Contemporary
Laser Dentistry

Anuj Singh Parihar

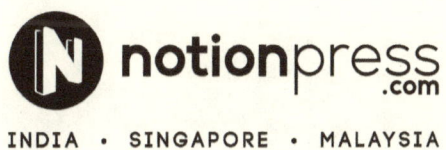

INDIA • SINGAPORE • MALAYSIA

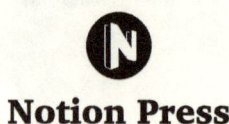

Notion Press

Old No. 38, New No. 6
McNichols Road, Chetpet
Chennai - 600 031

First Published by Notion Press 2018
Copyright © Anuj Singh Parihar 2018
All Rights Reserved.

ISBN 978-1-64324-704-5

This book has been published with all efforts taken to make the material error-free after the consent of the author. However, the author and the publisher do not assume and hereby disclaim any liability to any party for any loss, damage, or disruption caused by errors or omissions, whether such errors or omissions result from negligence, accident, or any other cause.

No part of this book may be used, reproduced in any manner whatsoever without written permission from the author, except in the case of brief quotations embodied in critical articles and reviews.

CONTENTS

Preface   *v*

Acknowledgements   *vii*

1. Introduction   1
2. History of Lasers   5
3. Electromagnetic Radiation and Electromagnetic Spectrum   11
4. Principles of Working of Lasers   13
5. Generation of Laser Energy   18
6. Classifications of Lasers   26
7. Types of Lasers   32
8. Properties of Laser Light   34
9. Photobiology of Lasers   38
10. Applications of Lasers   43
11. Current and Potential Applications of Lasers in Dentistry   45
12. Applications of Lasers in Periodontology   48
13. Applications of Lasers in Endodontics   63
14. Applications of Lasers in Oral Medicine   71

15.	Applications of Lasers in Orthodontics	77
16.	Applications of Lasers in Prosthodontics	85
17.	Recent Advances in Lasers	91
18.	Hazards of Lasers	92
19.	Laser Safety and Precautions	99
20.	Laser Safety Considerations in Dentistry	101
21.	Advantages and Disadvantages of Lasers	104
22.	Summary and Conclusion	105

References *107*

PREFACE

"Life is divided into three terms – that which was, which is, and which will be. Let us learn from the past to profit by the present, and from the present to live better in the future."

– **William Wordsworth**

This book has been written to meet the requirement of all individuals, from dental students to educators, clinicians to researchers and from specialists to generalists who want to understand and adapt lasers in their daily dental practice. Since last one decade, the use of lasers in dental practice has increased tremendously, a need has been felt for a book on this subject with quintessential content. A keen attempt has been made to make the book useful and interesting. Leaving aside all the unnecessary things, only the essential facts have been discussed in this book. It has a direct link with practical understanding, that all the hazards, disadvantages of lasers have been explained very clearly.

It has been experienced that newly graduated dentists who have opened their private practice lack in their confidence to use lasers at their work place. Therefore, this book has been written in such a way that it may equip the clinicians with through understanding about the lasers.

Any suggestions towards its further improvement will be thankfully acknowledged and incorporated in the next edition.

– **Anuj Singh Parihar**

ACKNOWLEDGEMENTS

"ALL Men like to think they can do it alone, but reality is, there is no substitute for support, encouragement or a fellow."

– **Tim Allen**

This and any other piece of work or activities that I have ever been able to reach is solely the blessings of my dearest parents, Shri. K.S. Parihar and my mother Smt. Bina Parihar. I am indebted for their love and blessings, for their continuous encouragement rendered throughout life and without which I would not have reached so far. Thank you for your unconditional support with my studies and every single pursuit in my life. I am honoured to have you as my parents.

I also like to thank my brother, Shri. Ankit Parihar (Manu), for always cheering and supporting me. Amongst friends, Dr. Parag Bhave and Dr. Lavanya Bhatnagar have assisted me and provided me with wonderful motivations.

Finally, I would like to thank my students for their unconditional love and respect which have been the source of my strength and motivation.

– **Anuj Singh Parihar**

INTRODUCTION

Lasers play a pivotal role in our day to day life. In fact they show up in an amazing range of products and technologies. One can find them in many things ranging from CD players to high-speed metal cutting machines to measuring systems tattoo removal, hair replacement, eye surgery etc.

The word LASER is an acronym for Light Amplification by Stimulated Emission of Radiation. Lasers have come down a long way since Albert Einstein described the theory of stimulated emission in 1917[1]. In 1953, Charles Hard Townes and graduate students James P. Gordon and Herbert J. Zeiger produced the first microwave amplifier, a device operating on similar principles to the laser, but amplifying microwave radiation rather than infrared or visible radiation. They called it Maser: "Microwave Amplification by Stimulated Emission of Radiation." In 1957, Charles Hard Townes and Arthur Leonard Schawlow, then at Bell Labs, began a serious study of the infrared laser. As ideas developed, they abandoned infrared radiation to instead concentrate upon visible light. The concept originally was called an "optical maser." In 1958, Bell Labs filed a patent application for their proposed optical maser; and Schawlow and Townes submitted a manuscript of their theoretical calculations to the *Physical Review*, published that year. Theodore Maiman in 1960, demonstrated Laser function with the use of a pink ruby crystal (sapphire with trivalent chromium impurities), optically pumped by a helical flashlamp that surrounded the cylindrical laser crystal. The parallel ends of the ruby crystal were silvered, with a small hole at one end for observing the radiation. The reflective surfaces comprised the optical resonator.

The output wavelength was 694 nm. It was T. Maiman who coined the name "laser," in analogy to maser, as an abbreviation of Light Amplification by Stimulated Emission of Radiation.[2]

The discovery of the ruby laser triggered an intensive search for other materials, and in rapid succession laser action in other solids, gases, semiconductors, and liquids was demonstrated. Following the discovery of the ruby laser, the next solid-state material was uranium-doped calcium fluoride which was lased in late 1960. The first solid-state neodymium laser was calcium tungstate doped with neodymium ions. This laser, discovered in 1961, was used in research facilities for a number of years until yttrium aluminate garnet, as a host material for neodymium, was discovered.[2]

The application of solid-state lasers for military tactical systems proceeded along a clear path since there is no alternative for rangefinders, target illuminators, and designators. At the same time construction of large Nd: glass lasers began at many research facilities. Also solid-state lasers were readily accepted as versatile research tools in many laboratories.

Much more difficult and rather disappointing at first was the acceptance of the solid-state lasers for industrial and medical applications. Despite improvement in systems reliability and performance, it took more than two decades of development and engineering improvements before solid-state lasers moved in any numbers out of the laboratory and onto the production floor or into instruments used in medical procedures. Often applications that showed technical feasibility in the laboratory were not suitable for production because of economic reasons, such as high operating costs or limited processing speeds. Also, other laser systems provided strong competition for a relatively small market. The CO_2 laser proved to be a simpler and more robust system for many industrial and medical applications.[2]

Several medical specialties use lasers in their daily practice, and it has become the standard of care for surgical therapy in ophthalmology, otolaryngology and gynecology, just to mention a few.[3]

For a laser to be useful in clinical practice, it must be able to effectively deliver laser energy to the target site. Early delivery systems were too bulky or cumbersome to use in the oral cavity. Today fiber optic delivery systems are the system of choice for most lasers as they can deliver laser energy to most parts of the oral cavity and even within the complex root canal system.[4]

The principle mechanism of action of laser energy on tissue is photothermal. The other mechanisms like ablastion in which rapid heating of water molecules within enamel causes rapid vaporization of the water and buildup of steam which causes an expansion that ultimately over comes the crystal strength of the dental structures, and the material breaks by exploding, may be secondary to this process. For a laser to have biological effect, the energy must be absorbed. The degree of absorption in tissue will vary as a function of the wavelength and optical characteristics of the target tissue.[4]

The recent rapid development of lasers, with different wavelengths and onboard parameters may continue to have major impact on the scope and practice of dentistry.

The use of lasers in dentistry has increased over the past few years. The first laser was introduced into the fields of medicine and dentistry during the 1960s (Goldman *et al.*, 1964). Since then, this science has progressed rapidly. Because of their many advantages, lasers are indicated for a wide variety of procedures (Frentzen and Koort, 1990; Aoki *et al.*, 1994; Pelagalli *et al.*, 1997; Walsh, 2003). It was Stern and Sognnaes who in 1964 used the Ruby laser to vaporize enamel and dentin. Weichman and Johnson in 1971 were the first to use lasers in Endodontics.[4] Conventional methods of cavity preparation with low- and high-speed handpieces involve noise, uncomfortable vibrations and stress for patients. Although pain may be reduced by local anaesthesia, fear of the needle and of noise and vibration of mechanical preparation remains causes of discomfort. These disadvantages have led to a search for new techniques as potential alternatives for dental hard tissue removal. In periodontal therapy lasers are used for procedures like frenectomy, frenotomy, melanin depigmentation, gingival excision curettage, many mucogingival procedures etc.

It is important to remember that in practice of medicine and dentistry, it is the physicians and dentists who are prime determinants of the quality of health care and not the tools chosen to use. Lasers are wonderful tools when used by an experienced well trained physician and dentist.

The aim of this book is to describe the role, applications and scope of lasers in dentistry.

HISTORY OF LASERS

Historically, the search for lasers began as an extension of stimulated amplification techniques employed in the microwave region. Masers, coined from Microwave Amplification by Stimulated Emission of Radiation, served as sensitive preamplifiers in microwave receivers. In 1954 the first maser was built by C. Townes and utilized the inversion population between two molecular levels of ammonia to amplify radiation at a wavelength around 1.25 cm.[5]

In 1955 an optical excitation scheme for masers was simultaneously proposed by N. Bloembergen, A.M. Prokorov, and N.G. Basov. A few years later, masers were mostly built using optically pumped ruby crystals. In 1958 A. Schawlow and C. Townes proposed extending the maser principle to optical frequencies and the use of a Fabry–Perot resonator for feedback. However, they did not find a suitable material or the means of exciting it to the required degree of population inversion.[5]

This was accomplished by T. Maiman who built the first laser in 1960. It was a pink ruby crystal (sapphire with trivalent chromium impurities), optically pumped by a helical flashlamp that surrounded the cylindrical laser crystal. The parallel ends of the ruby crystal were silvered, with a small hole at one end for observing the radiation. The reflective surfaces comprised the optical resonator. The output wavelength was 694 nm. It was T. Maiman who coined the name "laser," in analogy to maser, as an abbreviation of Light Amplification by Stimulated Emission of Radiation.[5]

In early ruby laser systems the output consisted of a series of irregular spikes, stretching over the duration of the pump pulse. A key discovery made by R.W. Hellwarth in 1961 was a method called Q-switching for concentrating the output from the ruby laser into a single pulse. This Q-switch, which consisted of a cell filled with nitrobenzene, required very high voltages for Q-switching; it was soon replaced by spinning one of the resonator mirrors. A further refinement was the insertion of a spinning prism between the fixed mirrors of the resonator.

The earliest application of the laser was in active range-finding by measuring the time of flight of a laser pulse reflected from a target. Investigations in this direction started immediately after the discovery of the ruby laser. Four years later, fully militarized rangefinders containing a flashlamp-pulsed ruby laser with a spinning prism Q-switch went into production. For about 10 years ruby-based rangefinders were manufactured; afterward the ruby laser was replaced by the more efficient neodymium doped yttrium aluminum garnet (Nd:YAG) laser.

The discovery of the ruby laser triggered an intensive search for other materials, and in rapid succession laser action in other solids, gases, semiconductors, and liquids was demonstrated. Following the discovery of the ruby laser, the next solid-state material was uranium-doped calcium fluoride which was lased in late 1960. The first solid-state neodymium laser was calcium tungstate doped with neodymium ions. This laser, discovered in 1961, was used in research facilities for a number of years until yttrium aluminate garnet, as a host material for neodymium, was discovered.[5]

In 1961, E. Snitzer demonstrated the first neodymium glass laser. Since Nd: glass could be made in much larger dimensions and with better quality than ruby, it promised to deliver much higher energies. Large budgets have been devoted to the development and installation of huge Nd: glass laser systems which became the world-wide systems of choice for laser fusion research and weapons simulation. The most powerful of these systems, the NOVA laser, completed in 1985, produced 100 kJ of energy in a 2.5 ns pulse. Systems with energies ten times larger are currently under construction.[5]

Using a ruby laser, P.A. Franken demonstrated second harmonic generation in crystal quartz in 1961. In 1962 the idea of parametric amplification and generation of tunable light was conceived, and a few years later the first experiment demonstrating parametric gain was achieved. Commercial parametric oscillators based on lithium niobate were introduced in 1971.

The first optical fiber amplifier was demonstrated in 1963 using a 1 m long neodymium-doped glass fiber wrapped around a flashlamp. However, the concept received little attention until the 1980s when low-loss optical fibers became available and the fiber-optic communications industry explored these devices for amplification of signals. In 1964 the best choice of a host for neodymium ions, namely yttrium aluminum garnet (YAG), was discovered by J. Geusic. Since that time, Nd:YAG remains the most versatile and widely used active material for solid-state lasers. Nd:YAG has a low threshold which permits continuous operation, and the host crystal has good thermal, mechanical, and optical properties and can be grown with relative ease.[5]

At the end of the 1960s, continuously pumped Nd:YAG lasers with multihundred watts output power became commercially available. In 1965, a technique termed "mode-locking" was invented. By the end of the 1960s, most of the important inventions with regard to solidstate laser technology had been made. Nd:YAG and Nd: glass proved clearly superior over many other solid-state laser materials; short-pulse generation by means of Q-switching and mode-locking, as well as frequency conversion with harmonic generators and parametric oscillators, was well understood.[5]

To gain wider acceptance in manufacturing processes, the reliability of the laser systems needed improvement and the operation of the lasers had to be simplified. During the 1970s, efforts concentrated on engineering improvements, such as an increase in component and system lifetime and reliability. The early lasers often worked poorly and had severe reliability problems.

Despite improvement in systems reliability and performance, it took more than two decades of development and engineering improvements before solid-state lasers moved in any numbers out of the laboratory and onto the production floor or into instruments used in medical procedures. Chromium-doped fluoride crystals such as lithium strontium aluminum fluoride and lithium calcium aluminum fluoride are of interest because they can be pumped with laser diodes.[5]

In the late 1980s, the combination of broad band tunable lasers in combination with ultrafast modulation techniques, such as Kerr lens mode-locking, led to the development of mode-locked lasers with pulse widths on the order of femtoseconds. In the 1970s, diode lasers capable of continuous operation at room temperature were developed. In the mid-1980s, with the introduction of epitaxial processes and a greatly increased sophistication in the junction structure of GaAs devices, laser diodes became commercially available with output powers of several watts. These devices had sufficient power to render them useful for the pumping of Nd: YAG lasers.

As diode lasers became less expensive, these pump sources were incorporated into smaller commercial solid-state lasers. At this point, laser diode-pumped solid-state lasers began their rapid evolution that continues today.

In this historical perspective we could sketch only briefly those developments that had a profound impact on the technology of solid-state lasers. Laser emission has been obtained from hundreds of solid-state crystals and glasses. However, most of these lasers are of purely academic interest. There is a big difference between laser research and the commercial laser industry, and there are many reasons why certain lasers did not find their way into the market or disappeared quickly after their introduction. Most of the lasers that did not leave the laboratory were inefficient, low in power, difficult to operate or, simply, less practical to use than other already established systems. Likewise, many pump schemes, laser configurations, and resonator designs did not come into use because of their complexity and commensurate high manufacturing and assembly costs or their difficulty in maintaining performance.

Lasers were first employed in dentistry in hard tissue treatments, such as caries removal and cavity preparation, as a substitute for mechanical cutting and drilling. After the discovery of the ruby laser in 1960, Goldman and coworkers attempted caries removal in vitro using the ruby laser in 1964. Since then, many researchers have investigated the effects of various lasers such as the argon, CO_2, and Nd:YAG lasers on dental hard tissues and caries. The initial and most important stage of periodontal therapy is the nonsurgical mechanical debridement of periodontally diseased root surfaces. In 1965, Kinersly et al. had already reported the possibility of removing dental calculus by ruby laser. However, they warned that limiting the vaporization selectively to calculus without damaging the underlying tooth might present clinical problems.

The commonly used high power lasers CO_2 and Nd:YAG are capable of excellent soft tissue ablation, and have an adequate hemostatic effect. As such, these lasers have been generally approved for soft tissue management in periodontics and oral surgery. However, these lasers are not useful for treatment of the root surface or alveolar bone, due to carbonization of these tissues and major thermal side-effects on the target and surrounding tissues. Until the beginning of the 1990s, the use of laser systems in periodontal therapy was limited to soft tissue procedures, such as gingivectomy and frenectomy, as application to periodontal hard tissues had previously proved to be clinically unpromising.[5]

In the early and mid 1990s, scientific research was begun on root surface debridement and pocket curettage using an Nd:YAG laser. Meanwhile, in 1988, Hibst et al. and, in 1989, Keller & Hibst and Kayano et al. reported the possibility of dental hard tissue ablation by Er:YAG laser irradiation, which is highly absorbed by water. Since then, numerous studies on hard tissue treatment using the Er: YAG laser have indicated the ability of this laser to ablate dental hard tissues and caries lesions without producing major thermal side-effects.[5]

Later, in the mid 1990s, Aoki et al. and Keller et al. began to investigate the application of the Er:YAG laser for periodontal hard tissue procedures, such as dental calculus removal and decontamination of the diseased root surface. A number of basic studies on Er:YAG laser application to root surface treatment followed and, recently, promising results have been reported in clinical studies on nonsurgical pocket therapy. Application of the Er:YAG laser for bone surgery has been also studied in vitro and in vivo. Development of this laser brought the prospect of hard tissue treatment in periodontics and endodontics, as well as in operative dentistry including pediatric dentistry.

The diode lasers as well as Nd:YAG lasers are currently used for pocket curettage by clinicians because of their flexible fiber delivery system, which is suitable for pocket insertion. However, to date, there is a shortage of basic and clinical research providing scientific support for these procedures.

In the field of dentistry, Nd:YAG, CO_2, diodes, Er:YAG, Er, Cr:YSGG, Argon, excimer and alexandrite lasers are being studied in vitro or are in clinical use. Their use in the treatment of periodontal pockets and/or debridement of the periodontally diseased root surface is presently under investigation.

ELECTROMAGNETIC RADIATION AND ELECTROMAGNETIC SPECTRUM

Electromagnetic radiation is the movement of energy through space as a combination of electric and magnetic fields. It is generated when the velocity of an electrically charged particle is altered. Electromagnetic spectrum is the orderly distribution of electromagnetic radiations in accordance with their wavelength or frequency. The classification of EM waves in the Electromagnetic spectrum do not have sharp boundaries as it is done according to its main source, and different sources may produce waves in overlapping ranges of frequency[6]. Although, summarizing the EM spectrum, we may classify it as:

1. Radio Frequency waves
2. Microwaves
3. Infrared radiations
4. Visible Spectrum
5. Ultraviolet rays
6. X-rays
7. Gamma Rays

Generally, Lasers function in so called optical spectrum, but depending upon the type and source of laser its wavelength ranges from the ultraviolet radiation to far Infrared region.[6]

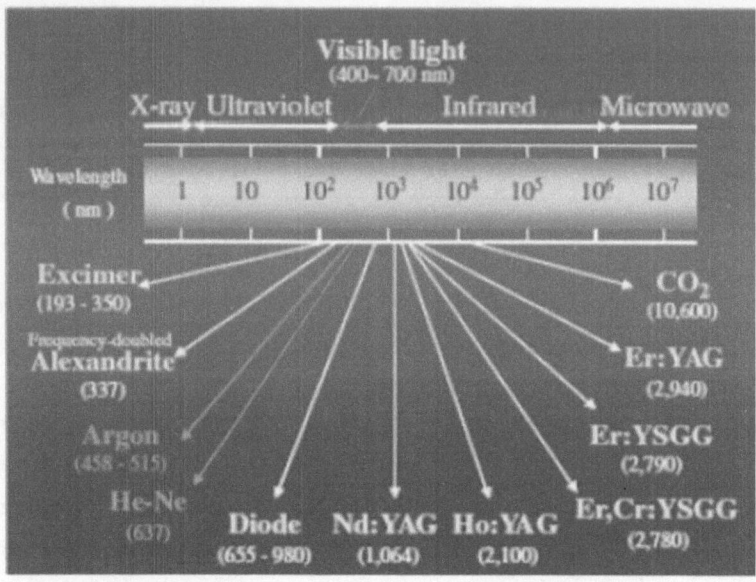

Fig. 1: The accepted Electromagnetic spectrum: All lasers represented on the EM spectrum depending on their specific wavelength.

PRINCIPLES OF WORKING OF LASERS

Interaction of Radiation with Matter: Quantum Mechanical View

The understanding of the principle of a laser requires an appreciation of quantum processes that takes place in a material when it is exposed to radiation. A material medium is composed of identical atoms or molecules each of which is characterized by a set of discrete allowed energy states. An atom can move from one energy state to another when it receives or releases an amount of energy. This energy is equal to the amount of energy difference between the two states. It is termed a quantum jump or transition. The interaction of radiation with atoms leads to the following three distinct competing processes in the medium.[6]

1. Absorption
2. Spontaneous Emission
3. Stimulated Emission

Absorption

An atom residing in the lower energy state may absorb the incident photon and jump to exited state. The transition is known as stimulated absorption or induced absorption or simply absorption. Corresponding to each transition made by an atom one photon disappears from the incident beam.[6]

Spontaneous Emission

Excited state with higher energy is inherently unstable because of a natural tendency of atoms to seek out the lowest energy configuration. Therefore, excited atoms do not stay in the excited state for a relatively longer time but tend to return to the lower state by giving up the excess energy in the form of spontaneous emission or stimulated emission. When this emission is on its own out of its natural tendency to attain minimum potential energy condition and without any external impetus, it is called as spontaneous emission.

The instant of the transition, direction of the emission of photon, the phase of the photon, the polarization of the photon are all random quantities. There will not exist any correlation among the parameters of the innumerable photons emitted spontaneously by the assembly of the atoms of the medium. Therefore, the light generated by the medium will be incoherent. It contains a superposition of many waves of random phases. The net intensity of such incoherent waves in proportional to the number of radiating atoms. The light is radiated in the form of short duration wave trains emitted in all directions and the intensity goes on decreasing as the wave trains travel away from the source. Each of them bears no consistent phase relationship with each other nor do they share common polarization plane. As a consequence, there is no compounding of the individual wave. The light is not monochromatic because of various line broadening processes that takes place in the medium.[6]

Stimulated Emission

An atom in the excited state need not wait for spontaneous emission to occur. There exists an alternative mechanism by which an excited atom can make a downward transition and emit light. A photon of similar energy can induce the excited atom to make a downward transition releasing the energy in the form of a photon. Thus the interaction of a photon with the excited atom triggers the excited atom to drop to the lower energy state up a photon. The phenomenon of emission of photon is called induced emission or stimulated emission. The existence of the mechanism was predicted by Einstein in 1916.

The process of stimulated emission is characterized by some very interesting features:

1. The emitted photon is identical to the incident photon in all respects. It has the same frequency as that of incident photon. It will be in phase with the incident photon. Both the photons travel in the same direction. They will be in the same state of polarization.
2. The process is controllable from outside.
3. The most important feature is that multiplication of photons takes place in the process. One photon induces an atom to emit a second photon, these two travelling along the same direction de-excite two atoms in their path producing a total of four photons which builds up in an avalanche like manner. It suggests that electromagnetic waves of extremely high amplitude could be generated by the combined stimulated emissions from large sample of atoms leading to amplification of light. The constructive interference of many waves travelling in the same direction with a common frequency and common phase produces an intense coherent light beam. The resultant light is a single plane wave in which all of the individual waves emitted by individual atoms have combined in phase. The net intensity is proportional to the number of atoms that contributed to it and the net intensity is proportional the square of the number of atoms. Since the number of atoms in light source is large, coherent emission leads to an enormous high intense light than incoherent emission. Therefore, the process of stimulated emission is the key to the operation of laser.[6]

Active Medium

A medium in which light gets amplified is called an active medium. The medium may be a solid, liquid or gas. Out of the different atoms in the medium, only a small fraction of atoms of particular species are responsible for stimulated emission and consequent light amplification. They are called active centers. The remaining bulk of the medium plays the role of host and supports active centers.[6]

Population Inversion

Laser operation requires obtaining stimulated emission almost exclusively. To achieve high percentage of stimulated emission, an artificial situation known as population inversion is to be created.

In a state of thermal equilibrium there are more atoms in lower level than in the upper level. There must be more atoms in the upper level than in the lower level in order to achieve stimulated emission exclusively. Therefore, a non-equilibrium state is to be produced in which the population of the upper energy level exceeds to a large extent the population of the lower energy level. When this situation occurs, the population distribution between the energy levels is said to be inverted, and the medium is said to have gone into the state of population inversion.[6]

Metastable State

An atom can be excited to a higher level by supplying energy to it. Normally, excited atoms have short lifetimes and release their energy in a matter of nanoseconds (10^{-9} s) through spontaneous emission. It means that the atoms do not stay long enough at the excited state to be stimulated. As a result, even though the pumping agent continuously raises the atoms to the excited level, they undergo spontaneous transitions and rapidly return to the lower energy level. Population inversion cannot be established under such circumstances. In order to establish the condition of the population inversion, the excited atoms are required to 'wait' at the upper energy level till a large number of atoms accumulate at that level. In other words, it is necessary that the excited state has a longer lifetime. A metastable state is such a state. Atoms excited to the metastable state remain excited for an appreciable time, which is of the order of 10^{-6} to 10^{-3}s. This is 10^3 to 10^6 times the lifetimes of the ordinary energy levels.

Therefore, the metastable state population can allow accumulation of a large number of excited atoms at that level. The metastable state population can exceed the population at a lower level and establish the condition of population inversion in the lasing medium. It would be impossible to create the state of system containing impurity atoms. These levels lie in the forbidden band gap of the host crystal. Population inversion readily takes place as the lifetime of these levels is large, and secondly, there is no competition in filling these levels, as they are localized levels.

There could be no population inversion and hence no laser action, if metastable states do not exist.[6]

GENERATION OF LASER ENERGY

The word laser is an acronym that actually names the device as well as the process by which laser radiation is generated. Laser, or Light Amplification by Stimulated Emission of Radiation, is a mnemonic term that describes the process in which a certain laser medium or lasant within a resonator space is energized by internal or external energy sources to produce an excited population of atoms, molecules, and rare gas (species). The energy within a resonator space reaches a population inversion in which the greatest cohort of species is in an excited state and in which photons are emitted and amplified within a laser cavity. The radiant energy is released as a laser beam.[6]

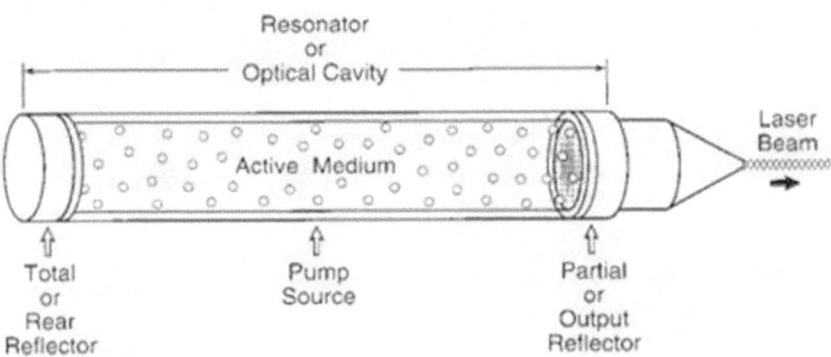

Fig. 2: The fundamental components of a laser. The lasant is composed of a laser medium consisting of a species that is the name of that laser. The species can consist of ions, atoms, and molecules.[6]

Fundamental Components of a Laser system

To understand the generation of laser radiation, it is probably expeditious to consider the fundamental design of the laser cavity, the system that houses the actual physical reaction that eventually results in the production of the laser beam. The fundamental components of a laser system include a resonant cavity housing an active medium that has the ability to produce a population inversion and energy input, either external or internal (Fig. 2). The active medium is housed by a cavity and bounded by two mirrors. These mirrors are designed to reflect photons completely on one end and partially on the other end of the cavity. Consequently, one end is completely reflective, and the other is semi-reflective and semitransparent to allow the radiant energy to exit the resonant cavity. Within the design of the laser device may be apertures to actually -shape the beam and shutters designed to control the power or magnitude of the energy and its periodicity. With the combination of two mirrors that are essentially parallel, the mirrors are placed at either end of the laser cavity consisting of for simplicity a cylinder.[6]

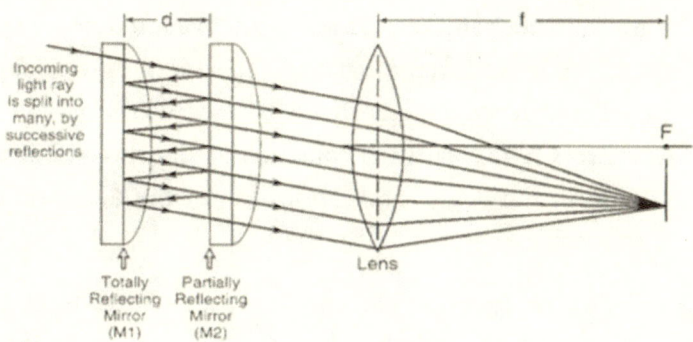

Fig. 3: The Fabry-Perot interferometer is made up of two mirrors M1 and M2, which are separated by a distance, d. Light of a given wavelength (gamma) after entering the interferometer will experience multiple reflections. Because mirror M2 is partially reflective, some light will pass out of the device. These light waves are then focused by the lens to a specific locus in the focal plane F, at which point interference takes place.[6]

The mirrors are separated by a fixed distance (d), forming a Fabry-Perot interferometer (Fig.3), which uses the physical principle of interference. Interference occurs when two or more waves simultaneously penetrate some material, forming a combined wave. The result is a larger wave having higher amplitude and thus deeper troughs. If these waves are in phase, they are said to be constructively interfering or exhibit constructive interference. Such light produced by constructive interference is brighter. The opposite can also occur, that is, destructive interference, in which the waves are not in phase. In such a case, the wave is of reduced amplitude and thus has less brightness. Indeed, if the two waves are of the same amplitude, the process of destructive interference means that the waves cancel and result in darkness. Light formed by laser action within the cavity from the active medium has a certain wavelength (A). The more the process of constructive interference occurs, the more consistent a wavelength is produced by the laser cavity. Photons of light travel a distance of 2d over each previous ray, which means that the distance is only 2d if the rays are perpendicular to the mirrors. Then constructive interference occurs if 2d is equal to mA, where m is an integer. Constructive interferences occur between all rays if the wavelength is equal to 2d/m (A = 2d/m). In this system, only certain wavelengths are consistent and result in constructive interference and thus a bright output. This critical factor means that a laser of a given length can emit light only of certain wavelengths that will fit within the resonant cavity formed by its mirrors. The concept of constructive/destructive interference is also paramount in the design and fabrication of the dielectric mirrors that are used in most laser systems (Fig. 4).[6]

The generation of laser radiant energy is singularly dependent on designing and forcing the light within the laser cavity to travel between the mirrors and be reflected theoretically infinitely through a process termed optical feedback (Fig. 5). One could conceive of the mirror system within the laser cavity as a completely silvered mirror opposed by a parallel partly silvered mirror that allows some light to leave the resonant cavity and to be emitted as a collimated beam of laser energy. The laser cavity is designed so that enough light reflects back into the laser complex, as are the dielectric mirrors, not only in their composition but also in their shape. It is not surprising that the mirrors forming the ends of the laser cavity are not the same kinds of mirrors that one would find in everyday use. Indeed, it is very difficult to maintain parallelism if one designs a laser based on parallel flat plane or so-called planar mirrors.[6]

Theoretically, one would have to continually adjust the mirrors for parallelism. Otherwise, a resonation of the beam to and fro would not occur and, indeed, amplification would be difficult.

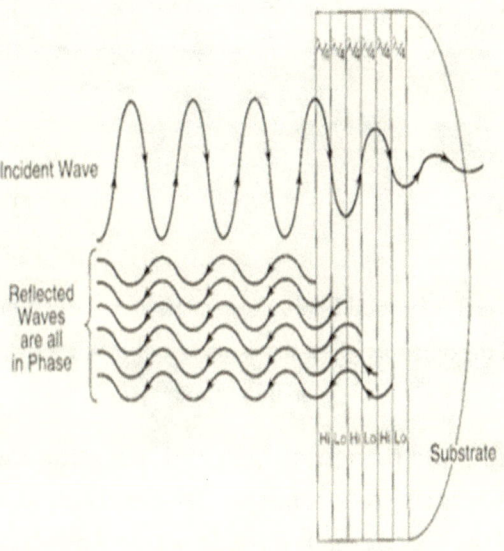

Fig. 4: This is a magnification of a section of the laser dielectric mirror. This shows an alternation of glasses of high (Hi) and low (Lo) refraction indices. By alternating the glasses as indicated, all reflections are forced to be in phase, resulting in a constructive interference and controlled reflectance.[6]

In lasers such as the argon laser, the minors are made of glass but do not have reflective surfaces as such. These mirrors are the dielectric mirrors, which rely on a constructive interference phenomenon to produce significant reflectivity. Within the dielectric system, there are alternative layers of high refractive index materials, such as titanium oxide, and low refractive index materials, such as silicon oxide (Fig. 4). Remarkably, these materials are deposited on a glass substrate and each layer is designed to be one quarter of a wavelength thick.[6]

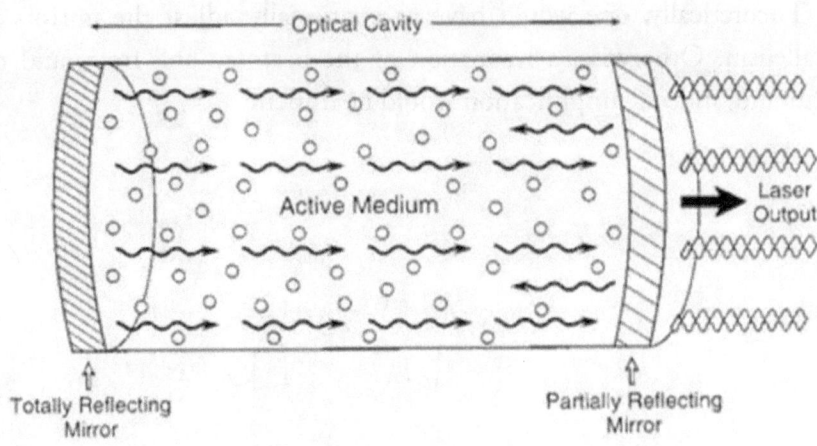

Fig. 5: A schematic of optical feedback in the laser chamber. One mirror is highly reflective, and the other permits a small amount of incident light to be released as useful output.[6]

By alternating the pattern of high and low refractive index materials, the light waves are reflected from successive surfaces and undergo a phase change equivalent to one half wavelength or 180 degrees on reflection from high-index materials. No phase change occurs on reflection from low-index materials; thus, the result is that all reflected rays are interfered with constructively, and light of this particular wavelength is kept inside the laser cavity, causing stimulated emission only at a specific controlled wavelength. The resulting waves that do not constructively interfere leak out of the system, and therefore, stimulated emission does not occur at those wavelengths. This alternating pattern results in all reflections that are in phase, causing constructive interference and a controlled reflectance from the mirror. Depending on the number of layers within the mirror, a direct linear relationship is observed with a number of layers. Consequently, as the number of layers increases up to 20 or more, the reflectance will approach 100% for at least one particular wavelength, as in a gas laser. One mirror is nearly a perfect reflector, and the other is 99% reflective, resulting in 1% of light at the desired wavelength emerging as the incident laser beam.[6]

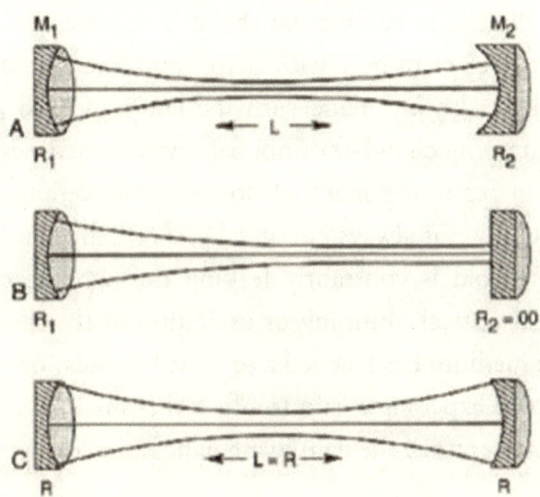

Fig. 6: Examples of curved mirror cavities: *A*, general form; B curved/plane shape; and C, confocal resonator. (L, Length of the laser cavity; M1 totally reflecting mirror; M2, partially reflecting mirror; R1 and R2, differing radii of curvature of the mirrors of M1 and M2. These radii determine the shape and dimensions of the laser beam. As one can see from the diagram, changes in the radius of curvature offers different beam patterns.

In C, the length of the laser cavity is equal to the radius of curvature or equal to the diameter of a circle represented by the radius of R; in this case, R = R.)[6]

Most medical and surgical lasers are not designed to operate with the plane parallel mirror system. These systems of planar mirror cavities are prone to small mal-alignment and also they will produce a poorly controlled beam shape. In the planar system, there is no specific axis that most photons would be forced to resonate upon so that, theoretically, the laser beam could resonate along several disparate axes, causing output that is spotty and randomly changing in-time. It is much more efficient to produce a curved mirror cavity, such as the curved planar configuration or the confocal resonator (Fig. 6). The actual optical cavity itself can be of many different shapes and materials. The simplest design is set up with one of the mirrors (M1) having a reflectivity of 100%, and the other (M2) having a reflectivity of less than 1% to 10%, which are called the total reflector and the output coupler, respectively. One can imagine an optical cavity with a cylindric or rectangular shape. There are also elliptic optical cavities or pumping chambers with a rod and lamp at the ellipse foci. Circular chambers also are made with the lamp and rod parallel to one another. The pumping chamber or optical cavity sometimes is constructed of a reflecting or scattering material, for example, ceramic or a polished metal. It is certainly not always circular. Weaker light that is not optically pumped to threshold is constantly leaking through the output coupler M2. However, if optical pumping or excitation of the species within the cavity or active medium has reached a so-called population inversion, then the light wave will experience gain to offset this small loss. The beam will gradually get weaker until the gain just balances the loss.[6]

If, for example, the total reflector and the output coupler equal 100% and 1%, respectively, then the light wave would have to increase by 1% in passing through the laser cavity or rod twice to just balance the 1% loss through the output coupler and out of the cavity. As alluded to earlier, the gain just equal to the loss is called the laser threshold. If the excitation increases or optical pumping of the active medium is enhanced above the threshold, this gives rise to a rapid increase in the beam power. In any laser cavity, only specific wavelengths will be capable of resonation as they reflect back and forth between the mirrors. A prerequisite to ensure resonance, and therefore, constructive interference and thus amplification, is that the length of the cavity should be a whole number of half wavelengths. That is to say, because $L = n \times$ the fraction $\lambda/2$ (where L is the length of the laser cavity and n is an integer), one can then use the equation that the frequency times the wavelength ($f\lambda$) is equal to the speed of light and reformatting $f = \lambda c/2L$. The frequencies within the laser cavity thus established are known as the cavity modes or, more clearly, the axial modes of the cavity. The cavity is extraordinarily long with regard to the actual wavelength of the emitted light from the active medium. The quantity n is thus an extraordinarily large number approximately 10^6, with a frequency difference between adjacent modes (known as the mode spacing) that is relatively small within the value of the order of several hundred megahertz (MHz).[6]

CLASSIFICATIONS OF LASERS

Lasers have been classified by wavelength and maximum output power into four classes and a few subclasses since the early 1970s. The classifications categorize lasers according to their ability to produce damage in exposed people, from class 1 (no hazard during normal use) to class 4 (severe hazard for eyes and skin). There are two classification systems, the "old system" used before 2002, and the "revised system" being phased in since 2002. The latter reflects the greater knowledge of lasers that has been accumulated since the original classification system was devised, and permits certain types of lasers to be recognized as having a lower hazard than was implied by their placement in the original classification system. The revised system is part of the revised IEC 60825 standard. From 2007, the revised system is also incorporated into the US-oriented ANSI Laser Safety Standard (ANSI Z136.1).[2]

The classification of a laser is based on the concept of *accessible emission limits* (AEL) that are defined for each laser class. This is usually a maximum power (in W) or energy (in J) that can be emitted in a specified wavelength range and exposure time that passes through a specified aperture stop at a specified distance. For infrared wavelengths above 4 μm, it is specified as a maximum power density (in W/m^2).[2]

Old System

The safety classes in the "old system" of classification were established in the United Statesthrough consensus standards (ANSI Z136.1) and Federal and state regulations. The international classification described in consensus standards such as IEC 825 (later IEC 60825) was based on the same concepts but presented with designations slightly different from the US classification.[2]

This classification system is only slightly altered from the original system developed in the early 1970s. It is still used by US laser product safety regulations. The laser powers mentioned are typical values. Classification is also dependent on the wavelength and on whether the laser is pulsed or continuous.[2]

Class I

Inherently safe; no possibility of eye damage. This can be either because of a low output power (in which case eye damage is impossible even after hours of exposure), or due to an enclosure preventing user access to the laser beam during normal operation, such as in CD players or laser printers.[2]

Class II

The blink reflex of the human eye (aversion response) will prevent eye damage, unless the person deliberately stares into the beam for an extended period. Output power may be up to 1 mW. This class includes only lasers that emit visible light. Most laser pointers are in this category.[2]

Class IIa

A region in the low-power end of Class II where the laser requires in excess of 1000 seconds of continuous viewing to produce a burn to the retina. Commercial laser scanners are in this subclass.[2]

Class IIIa

Lasers in this class are mostly dangerous in combination with optical instruments which change the beam diameter or power density, though even without optical instrument enhancement direct contact with the eye for over two minutes may cause serious damage to the retina.

Output power does not exceed 5 mW. Beam power density may not exceed 2.5 mW/square cm if the device is labeled with a "caution" warning label, otherwise a "danger" warning label is required. Many laser sights for firearms and laser pointers are in this category.[2]

Class IIIb

Lasers in this class may cause damage if the beam enters the eye directly. This generally applies to lasers powered from 5–500 mW. Lasers in this category can cause permanent eye damage with exposures of 1/100th of a second or less depending on the strength of the laser. A diffuse reflection is generally not hazardous but specular reflections can be just as dangerous as direct exposures. Protective eyewear is recommended when direct beam viewing of Class IIIb lasers may occur. Lasers at the high power end of this class may also present a fire hazard and can lightly burn skin. Many "laser pointers" at this output level are now available in this category.[2]

Class IV

Lasers in this class have output powers of more than 500 mW in the beam and may cause severe, permanent damage to eye or skin without being magnified by optics of eye or instrumentation. Diffuse reflections of the laser beam can be hazardous to skin or eye within the Nominal Hazard Zone. Most industrial, scientific, military, medical, and some hand held lasers are in this category.[2]

REVISED SYSTEM

Below, the main characteristics and requirements for the classification system as specified by the IEC 60825-1 standard are listed, along with typical required warning labels. Additionally, classes 2 and higher must have the triangular warning label and other labels are required in specific cases indicating laser emission, laser apertures, skin hazards, and invisible wavelengths.[2]

Class 1

A Class 1 laser is safe under all conditions of normal use. This means the maximum permissible exposure (MPE) cannot be exceeded when viewing a laser with the naked eye or with the aid of typical magnifying optics (e.g. telescope or microscope). To verify compliance, the standard specifies the aperture and distance corresponding to the naked eye, a typical telescope viewing a collimated beam, and a typical microscope viewing a divergent beam. It is important to realize that certain lasers classified as Class 1 may still pose a hazard when viewed with a telescope or microscope of sufficiently large aperture.[2]

Class 1M

A Class 1M laser is safe for all conditions of use except when passed through magnifying optics such as microscopes and telescopes. Class 1M lasers produce large-diameter beams, or beams that are divergent. The MPE for a Class 1M laser cannot normally be exceeded unless focusing or imaging optics are used to narrow the beam. If the beam is refocused, the hazard of Class 1M lasers may be increased and the product class may be changed. A laser can be classified as Class 1M if the power that can pass through the pupil of the naked eye is less than the AEL for Class 1, but the power that can be collected into the eye by typical magnifying optics (as defined in the standard) is higher than the AEL for Class 1 and lower than the AEL for Class 3B.[2]

Class 2

A Class 2 laser is safe because the blink reflex will limit the exposure to no more than 0.25 seconds. It only applies to visible-light lasers (400–700 nm). Class-2 lasers are limited to 1 mW continuous wave, or more if the emission time is less than 0.25 seconds or if the light is not spatially coherent. Intentional suppression of the blink reflex could lead to eye injury. Many laser pointers and measuring instruments are class 2.[2]

Class 2M

A Class 2M laser is safe because of the blink reflex if not viewed through optical instruments. As with class 1M, this applies to laser beams with a large diameter or large divergence, for which the amount of light passing through the pupil cannot exceed the limits for class 2.[2]

Class 3R

A Class 3R laser is considered safe if handled carefully, with restricted beam viewing. With a class 3R laser, the MPE can be exceeded, but with a low risk of injury. Visible continuous lasers in Class 3R are limited to 5 mW. For other wavelengths and for pulsed lasers, other limits apply.[2]

Class 3B

A Class 3B laser is hazardous if the eye is exposed directly, but diffuse reflections such as those from paper or other matte surfaces are not harmful. The AEL for continuous lasers in the wavelength range from 315 nm to far infrared is 0.5 W. For pulsed lasers between 400 and 700 nm, the AEL is 30 mW. Other limits apply to other wavelengths and to ultrashort pulsed lasers. Protective eyewear is typically required where direct viewing of a class 3B laser beam may occur. Class-3B lasers must be equipped with a key switch and a safety interlock.[2]

Class 4

Class 4 is the highest and most dangerous class of laser, including all lasers that exceed the Class 3B AEL. By definition, a class 4 laser can burn the skin, or cause devastating and permanent eye damage as a result of direct, diffuse or indirect beam viewing. These lasers may ignite combustible materials, and thus may represent a fire risk. These hazards may also apply to indirect or non-specular reflections of the beam, even from apparently matte surfaces—meaning that great care must be taken to control the beam path. Class 4 lasers must be equipped with a key switch and a safety interlock. Most industrial, scientific, military, and medical lasers are in this category, notably those at the US National Ignition Facility or at the UK Central Laser Facility.[2]

TYPES OF LASERS

There are many different types of lasers. The laser medium can be a solid, gas, liquid or semiconductor. Lasers are commonly designated by the type of lasing material employed.[2]

- **Solid-State Lasers** have lasing material distributed in a solid matrix (such as the ruby or neodymium: yttrium-aluminum garnet "Yag" lasers). The neodymium-Yag laser emits infrared light at 1,064 nanometers (nm).

- **Gas lasers** (helium and helium-neon, He–Ne, are the most common gas lasers) have a primary output of visible red light. CO_2 lasers emit energy in the far infrared, and are used for cutting hard materials.

- **Excimer lasers** (the name is derived from the terms excited and dimers) use reactive gases, such as chlorine and fluorine, mixed with inert gases such as argon, krypton or xenon. When electrically stimulated, a pseudo molecule (dimer) is produced. When lased, the dimer produces light in the ultra violet range.

- **Dye lasers** use complex organic dyes, such as rhodamine 6G, in liquid solution or suspension as lasing media. They are tunable over a broad range of wavelengths.

- **Semiconductor lasers,** sometimes called diode lasers, are not solid-state lasers. These electronic devices are generally very small and use low power. They may be built into larger arrays, such as the writing source in some laser printers or CD players.[2]

Table 1: Types of lasers with different wavelengths used in clinical dentistry[7]

Type	Active Medium	Wavelength (nm)
Gas laser	Carbon Dioxide (CO_2)	10,600
Diode lasers	Indium- Gallium Arsenide Phosphide (InGaAsP) Gallium Aluminium Arsenide (GaAlAs) Gallium- Arsenide (GaAs)	655-810-980
Solid-state Lasers	Neodymium doped: Yittrium Aluminium Garnet (Nd:YAG)	1,064
	Erbium doped: Yittrium Aluminium Garnet (Er:YAG)	2,940
	Erbium Chromium doped: Yittrium Selenium Gallium-Garnet (Er,Cr:YSGG)	2,780

PROPERTIES OF LASER LIGHT

There are several important properties of laser light that distinguish it from white light. These singular properties of laser light that make it useful for surgery are monochromaticity, directionality, coherence, and brightness. For over two centuries, there has been controversy surrounding the precise physical character of light or EM radiation. Light can be viewed both as a particle and as a wave, and behaves as both in certain physical instances. A light wave can be thought of as a stone dropped into a pool of water. The wave that radiates away from the impact point has an amplitude, frequency, and wavelength. The peak of the wave or its vertical height is called the amplitude, and this is related analogously to the intensity of a light wave. The number of wave peaks per second passing a specific static measuring point is the frequency of the wave expressed in light as hertz. Measuring the distance from one peak to the trough is called the wavelength. In light radiation, the wavelength and frequency determine the actual energy level of light and how it is distinguished or positioned within the EM spectrum. Longer wavelengths in the EM spectrum such as infrared, produce lower energy, and they include not only infrared but microwaves, television waves, and radio waves. Shorter wavelengths have higher energy and include ultraviolet, x-ray, and gamma radiation.[6]

Laser radiation is an intense beam of light that generates energy in the wavelengths that range from the near-ultraviolet to the near-infrared frequencies. The energy thus generated by a laser beam and its position within the EM spectrum are determined by the wavelength and frequency of the light wave. Whether or not the laser light is visible or invisible to the human eye depends on the medium used to generate laser light, the lasant. The carbon dioxide, Nd:YAG, helium-neon (HeNe), argon, and holmium: YAG lasers are of current interest and value to the oral and maxillofacial surgeon. The method by which radiation is generated from these systems is of clinical importance to the surgeon and will be discussed further.[6]

The notion that light is composed of packets of independent energy units was advanced by Sir Isaac Newton. Much later in the 20th century, the concept of quanta was used by Neils Bohr and Einstein to reconcile the concept that light was composed of packets of energy. Later, Einstein proposed the concept that light emanates in currents of massless particles referred to as photons, each photon carrying a specific quantum of energy and associated with a specific wavelength. This is the accepted theory and terminology used in laser physics. However, neither the wave concept nor the particulate concept fully explains all of the properties and observations of radiant light and other forms of EM radiation.

Monochromaticity

Lasers emit light that is monochromatic or specifically a single wavelength. This contrasts greatly with a typical incandescent light bulb, which emits colors of the entire spectrum, usually wavelengths from ultraviolet through the entire visible and then into the infrared range of 500 nm or more. An example of monochromaticity is the ability of a laser to selectively destroy tumor cells that have absorbed a particular dye such as hematoporphyrin derivative (HPD) or other tissue photosensitizer while not injuring contiguous or overlying cells. Lasers of varying types emit an individual wavelength or specified wavelengths, and indeed, some can be tuned to different wavelengths based on the desires of the operator. Importantly, each type of target tissue absorbs a given wavelength far better than others. This factor is based on the specific consistency of the tissue, its thickness, and significant tissue chromophores such as melanin and hemoglobin.[6]

Directionality

There is little divergence of the laser as it exits the laser device, and the beam can travel a considerable distance with very little movement away from parallelism. Most gas or solid-state lasers emit laser beams with a divergence angle of approximately a milliradian. In other words, they will spread out to one meter in diameter after traveling a kilometer. This also explains why laser light is extraordinarily hazardous. By not diverging over distance, laser light maintains brightness. For example, after traversing 10 meters across a large room, the beam could still be within a range of 10 mm across, still concentrated enough to be dangerous.[6]

Coherence

Coherence is a property of laser light that occurs when there is some fixed-phase relationship between two waves of laser light. There are two types of coherence of laser light, longitudinal and transverse. The longitudinal type of coherence represents a time or temporal coherence along the longitudinal beam axis, whereas transverse or spatial coherence refers to coherence across the beam. Thus, each wave is in phase with the other (Fig. 7). Both longitudinal and transverse coherence are produced by the process of stimulated emission and by resonation or optical feedback. Coherence thus causes the collimation of a laser beam over extremely large distances and allows the beam to accept extremely fine focusing. Any given laser beam can be focused only to a diameter equal to the wavelength of the specific laser. There is, of course, a finite coherent length or that distance over which the light produced is in actual phase; however, for conventional light sources, that distance is, for practical purposes.[6]

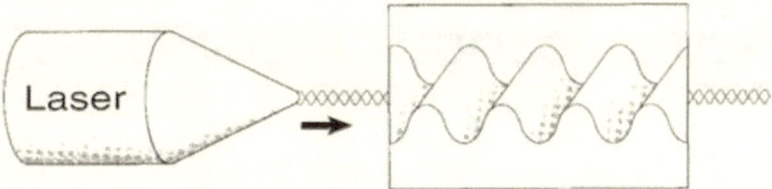

Fig. 7: Stimulated emission in which radiant photons move longitudinally along the axis of the laser chamber and stimulate other proximal excited atoms to also emit additional identical photons that will travel with the same directionality as the other stimulated photons within the laser chamber. This is the cascade phenomenon.[6]

Brightness

Another property of laser light that distinguishes it from conventional light sources, is that of brightness. This property arises from the parallelism or collimation of the laser light as it moves through space maintaining its concentration and, thus, the characteristic brightness. This high-brightness factor translates to high concentrations of energy when the laser is focused on a small spot. Conventional light sources can be focused, but the ultimate image is much larger than the microscopic focal spot of the laser beam. This focusing of the brightness of the laser beam is what the surgeon depends on to elevate the temperature of tissues or to cut or vaporize. Although there is dependence on defraction limitations, that is the focal spot can only equal the length of the specific laser wavelengths, there are instances in which the laser light can be concentrated microscopically to extremely high levels, resulting in atoms within the target zone becoming ionized as a result of the EM field energy's ability to strip electrons from the outer atomic shells and directly ionize the tissue. This forms a disruptive pattern referred to as optical plasma, and this pattern can be used to cut tissues and is useful in ophthalmology.[6]

PHOTOBIOLOGY OF LASERS

Tissue Effects of Laser Radiation

When radiant energy is absorbed by tissue: four basic types of interactions or responses can occur.

1. Photo chemical interaction
2. Photo thermal interaction
3. Photo mechanical interaction
4. Photo electrical interaction

Photochemical Interaction

The basic principle of the photochemical process is that specific wavelengths of laser lights are absorbing substances. A common example of a naturally occurring photochemical reaction is photosynthesis: where photons are absorbed by the chromophore, chlorophyll, to convert light energy into adenosine triphosphate (ATP).

$$6CO_2 + 6H_2O \xrightarrow[\text{Light energy}]{\text{Chlorophyll}} C_6H_{12}O_6 + 6O_2$$

Laser induced photochemical reactions such as tissue fluoresced phosphorescent re-emission may be used for diagnostic purposes.

Fluorescent tissue interaction or phosphorescent re-emission occurs when light energy is absorbed by specific molecules or tissue components that momentarily store and subsequently releases the energy again as light. The process of tissue florescence/phosphorescent remission is called photochemical decomposition.[6]

Photochemical interaction includes bio stimulation describing the stimulatory effects of laser light on biochemical and molecular process that normally occurs in tissues such as healing and repair.

Photo Thermal Interaction

Here radiant light energy absorbed by tissue substances and molecules becomes transformed into heat energy: which produces the tissue effect. The amount of laser light energy absorbed into tissue depends on a number of factors that include the wavelength of the radiant energy from the laser.

The laser parameter such as spot size; power density pulse duration and frequency and the optical properties and composition affect the target tissue. This class of interaction is the basis for most types of surgical laser application.

Because of its importance intensive research has been performed to identify biological response of the tissue. Tissue dehydration also plays a significant role in the thermal interaction of laser with tissue. Laser induced dehydration of tissue is a natural sequel of the heat generated within the thermally affected area.[6]

Photomechanical and Photoelectrical Stimulation

Photo disruption, photo disassociation, photoplasmolysis and photacoustic interactions are terms used to describe specific types of essentially non thermal process of laser tissue interactions. Photo disruption occurs whenever the photon energy of the incident beam exceeds either the atomic/molecular energies of the target tissue.

The process involved for photo disruption to occur can be divided into 3 interrelated mechanism phases 1) Ionization, 2) Plasma formation,

3) Shock wave generation. Ionization occurs in tissues at very high energy densities when the electric field strength of the beam becomes high enough to ionize atoms.

Once ionization occurs, a hot electrically charged gas of free electrons and positive ions, or plasma, is formed. As the temperature fluctuates within the electrical fluid from the laser, electrons within the plasma begins to vibrate, creating a rapid expansion and contraction that leads to generation of shock waves that can be heard as a sharp popping sound. Since it is a strong absorber of all wavelengths, the plasma act as shield, preventing further penetration of the beam to the target tissues.[6]

Clinical Manifestation of Laser Tissue Interactions Ablation and Incision

Removal of oral lesions by application of laser energy may be easily performed for surface exophytic and invasive lessons. The ablation of surface lesions by use of an unfocused beam of relatively large diameter (1 cm/greater) is easily accomplished through the effects of vaporization. Excision of xerophytes/invasive lesions may also be performed with a focused beam of 1mm or less to cut/incise tissues in a manner similar to that when a scalpel is used.[6]

Time Dependent Tissue Effects

The amount of transfer of radiant energy into thermal energy that occurs during absorption will be related to the power density of the incident radiation and duration of the exposure. The extent of tissue damage will be both power and time dependent. Hence reorganizing the different tissues among tissue type is also essential to establish suitable exposure parameter for the various types of tissue encountered in the oral cavity. Variations in water content in fibrous non-inflamed tissue and inflamed edematous tissues require consideration when selecting laser parameter to avoid excessive heating and charring of tissue during surgical procedure.[6]

Hemostasis, Sterlization and Tissue Welding

All these results from the thermal interaction of laser with biological tissue coagulation of blood and tissue proteins is the primary mechanism by which can occur. Irreversible damage to tissue in the form of coagulation or thermal necrosis of tissue inevitability accompanied the process of coagulation.

Homeostasis is thus possible with many laser systems through the heating of blood elements, and by direct sealing of small blood vessels by desiccation and contraction of the vessel wall.

Denaturation of serum and tissue proteins occurs at prolonged temperature of 65°C to 70°C. The welding of soft tissue by laser irradiation has been suggested as a potential method to replace suturing in some surgical applications. Tissue elements such as small blood vessels and tissue grafts may be joined together by an elevation from 70°C to 80°C. The process of tissue welding appears to be dependent on the denaturation of structural tissue proteins. Typically Argon, CO_2 and Nd:YAG lasers have been used by medical surgical specialties to weld nerves, small blood vessels and skins. Sterilization/disinfection of tissue surface has been described or additional benefits of laser use by a number of sources when laser are used to aveate tissue, the surface temperature is elevated to levels adequate to destroy microorganism. The antibacterial effect of CO_2 laser use in soft tissue surgery has been well established.[6]

Laser Energy and Tissue Temperature

The thermal effect of laser energy on soft tissue primarily revolves around the water content of the tissue and the temperature rise of the tissue. When the tissue temperature reaches approximately 60°C, proteins begin to denature without any vaporization of the underlying tissue. This phenomenon is useful in surgically removing diseased granulomatous tissue.

When the target tissue is elevated to a temperature of 100°C, vaporization of the water within the tissue occurs. Because of soft tissue water content, excision of soft tissue begins at this temperature. When the tissue temperature is raised to about 200°C, it is dehydrated, then burned and carbonization is the result. Carbon is a high absorber of all wavelengths so that the carbonized or charred tissue can become a heat sink as the lasing continues. The heat conduction then causes a great deal of collateral thermal damage to wide area.[6]

EFFECTS OF TEMPERATURE ON TARGET TISSUE

Tissue temperature (°C)	Observed effect
37–50	Hyperthermia
>60	coagulation, protein denaturation
70–90	Welding of tissue
>200	Carbonization

APPLICATIONS OF LASERS

Lasers are profitably used in almost every field. They are used in fundamental research. They are applied in entertainment electronics, industrial electronics, communications, mechanical working, machining, welding, surveying, astronomy, mechanical measurements, and information processing and even in warfare to guide missiles to the targets. The list is unending and continues to grow. Low power semiconductors are used in CD players, laser printing, copiers, range finders, strain gauges, optical micrometer. Very high power lasers are used to bring about thermonuclear reactions which would become the ultimate inexhaustible power source for human civilization. One of the important applications of laser is in the production of three dimensional images of an object in a process called holography.

The highly collimated beam of a laser can be further focused to a microscopic dot of extremely high energy density. This makes it useful as a cutting and cauterizing instrument. Lasers are used for photocoagulation of the retina to halt retinal hemorrhaging and for the tacking of retinal tears. Higher power lasers are used after cataract surgery if the supportive membrane surrounding the implanted lens becomes milky. Photodisruption of the membrane often can cause it to draw back like a shade, almost instantly restoring vision. A focused laser can act as an extremely sharp scalpel for delicate surgery, cauterizing as it cuts. ("Cauterizing" refers to long-standing medical practices of using a hot instrument or a high frequency electrical probe to singe the tissue around an incision, sealing off tiny blood vessels to stop bleeding.)

The cauterizing action is particularly important for surgical procedures in blood-rich tissue such as the liver.

Lasers have been used to make incisions half a micron wide, compared to about 80 microns for the diameter of a human hair.

CURRENT AND POTENTIAL APPLICATIONS OF LASERS IN DENTISTRY

Lasers for use in dentistry have been generally available for approximately two decades, with the first investigation of a dental laser having occurred more than forty years ago. The first laser using helium was created in 1960, and the first diode laser, which had a wavelength of 850 nm, was developed in 1962.[8]

Several types of laser systems are available, with some specific to either hard- or soft-tissue applications. Hard-tissue lasers are capable of treatment procedures for bone and tooth structure. Soft-tissue lasers are capable of treatment procedures for gingival tissues.

Hard Tissue Applications

Lasers for hard-tissue procedures are considerably larger and more expensive than lasers for soft-tissue procedures. Hard-tissue lasers, designed for the preparation of teeth, are limited to creating the cavity designs predicated by most direct restorative materials. Although very useful for conservative preparations, their use for more advanced cavity preparations for indirect restorations is limited and time-consuming. The Er:YAG dental laser first was approved for cavity preparation and caries removal in 1997.[8]

FDA (Food and Drug Administration) – Approved Hard Tissue Procedures[8]

- Removal of caries
- Cavity preparation
- Etching of enamel
- Enameloplasty, excavation of pits and fissures for placement of sealants
- Cutting, shaving, contouring, and resection of oral osseous tissue
- Apicoectomy
- Endodontics

Soft Tissue Applications

Soft-tissue procedures can be performed using lasers, electrosurgery units and scalpels. Each of these devices has advantages and disadvantages. The soft tissue lasers available are carbon dioxide lasers, Nd:YAG lasers, argon lasers, H:YAG lasers, Er,Cr:YSGG lasers and diode lasers; they differ in what is used to produce the energy, the wavelength of the light emitted from the laser, and whether the energy is supplied in a continuous or pulsed manner.[8]

Examples of soft-tissue lasers and wavelengths

- Carbon dioxide lasers 10,600 nm
- Er:YAG lasers 2,950 nm
- Er,Cr: YSGG lasers 2,780 run
- Nd:YAG lasers 1,064nm
- Diode lasers 810–980 nm
- Argon lasers 457–502nm

FDA (Food and Drug Administration) – Approved Soft Tissue Procedures[8]

- Abscess incision and drainage
- Biopsies (incisional/excision)

- Leukoplakia
- Aphthous ulcer treatment
- Crown lengthening (soft tissue only)
- Hemostatic assistance
- Fibroma removal
- Frenectomy
- Frenotomy
- Melanin depigmentation
- Gingival excision/incision
- Gingivectomy/gingivoplasty
- Operculectomy
- Oral papillectomy
- Tissue retraction for impression
- Vestibuloplasty
- Exposure of non-erupted or partially erupted teeth
- Implant recovery
- Lesion (tumor) removal
- Pulpotomy
- Pulpotomy as an adjunct to root canal therapy
- Removal of filling material, such as gutta percha or resin, as an adjunct treatment during root canal retreatrnent
- Sulcular debridement (removal of diseased or inflamed soft tissue in the periodontal pocket) to improve clinical indices, including gingival index, gingival bleeding index, probing pocket depth, attachment level, and tooth mobility.

APPLICATIONS OF LASERS IN PERIODONTOLOGY

The use of lasers for periodontal treatment becomes more complicated because the periodontium consists of both hard and soft tissues. Among the many lasers available, high power lasers such as CO_2, Nd:YAG and diode lasers can be used in periodontics because of their excellent soft tissue ablation and hemostatic characteristics. However, when they are applied to the root surface or alveolar bone, carbonisation and thermal damage have been reported. Therefore the use of these lasers is limited to gingivectomy, frenectomy and similar soft tissue procedures including the removal of melanin pigmentation of gingiva. Lasers are also used as an alternative or an adjunctive to conventional scaling and root debridement.

Removal of Calculus

- If a significant amount of calculus is present it must be removed to allow for sulcular access with the laser fiber.
- The power setting on the lasers are 10 to 20 pulses per second with 1.6 to 2w of energy.
- The fiber is passed through the sulcus of each tooth in slow sweeping movements, horizontally and vertically.[9]
- The patient then is placed on the proper maintenance schedule.

Bactericidal Effects of Lasers in Periodontal Pockets

The oral tissues readily absorb the blue green visible light of the argon, laser especially when pigmented with mealnin or haemoglobin. The argon wavelength is ideal for removal and cauterization of Hemangiomas and other pigmented highly vascular lesions. This characteristic has been used in the selective absorption of the argon laser energy by black pigmented bacteria. The gram-negative black pigmented anaerobes are the principal putative pathogens in the periodontal lesion.

Laser Pocket Thermolysis

This term has been used to describe the control of the pathogenic pocket Flora by argon laser energy in conjunction with scaling and root planning.[10]

- The laser tip is inserted into the pocket extending to the base and moved around the tooth circumferentially.
- The pathogens are colonized, as are the non-adherent plaque deposits and some of the adherent plaque on the root surface as well.
- Root instrumentation follows to remove the material from the pocket.
- This removal leaves a smooth root surface, which is compatible with healing on the soft tissue inflammatory lesion.
- Also CO_2 and Nd:YAG lasers are effective and adjunct with mechanical root instrumentation in the inflammatory control phase of periodontal therapy.
- Concomitant use of the laser during root instrumentation not only detoxifies the pocket but also removes the surface layer of microbial plaque from the underlying calculus and allows for easier effective root planning. The value of adjunctive lasing of the pocket is enhanced in bacterial reduction.[11]

Curettage

Curettage as a monotherapy for gain of attachment but generally has been discarded since 1989. Laser curettage in suprabony pockets where osseous surgery is not required when performed with mechanical root instrumentation is a considerably less invasive procedure. There is no evidence that traditional curettage/excisional new attachment procedure provides any significant differences in attachment gain. This procedure is accomplished with good hemostasis at low power setting and often precludes the need for anesthesia. Meyer noted that candidates for laser curettage are patients with periodontal pockets of 3 to 7 mm and it lasers the sulcus in a crisscross manner.[12]

The Nd:YAG laser with the 300 u fibers is inserted to the depth of the inflamed sulcus. Without anesthesia using a low power setting of 1.4W, the tip is moved slowly circumferentially around the tooth. This is followed by hand instrumentation. The clinical appearance 3 weeks later showed significant reduction of the inflammatory response, diminished probing depth and virtually no bleeding on probing. There is also evidence that laser assisted periodontal curettage is effective in preventing bacteremia before cardio vascular surgery.

Removal of Granulation Tissue

The CO_2 lasers can be used to remove granulation tissue either for periodontal "clean out," or for degranulating any wound site present. In certain furcation areas, circumferential defects, intrabony defects, and three wall defects, where stubborn tissue tags can persist, the laser can help either entirely to degranulate or partially degranulate these areas. Caution must be taken not to damage root surface or osseous structures. Carbon dioxide lasers with hollow wave guides are recommended for this purpose since the tip can be easily directed to the site to be degranulated. The laser should be used in the focused or near focused mode, and power settings should be adjusted from 1 to 2 W of indicated power with possible gating of the beam. When working in the areas of larger openings or better accessibility, higher power settings can be used but, again, with caution. Other wavelengths such as argon or Nd:YAG may prove to be more practical for this application.

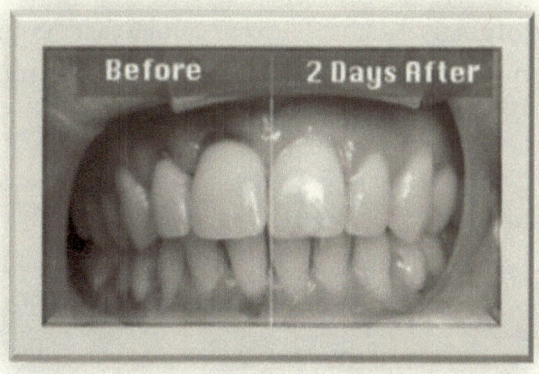

Fig. 8: Treatment of Chronic Periodontitis with Lasers

Gingivectomy and Gingivoplasty

These are carried our easily in a contact mode with pulsed or continuous wave lasers. The amount of anesthesia required is minimal and in some cases not necessary. The pulse duration of the Nd:YAG laser is 150 ms, which is apparently below the level of the removal action potential.

Pick (1985) described the laser gingivectomy as visual surgical procedure, when proper protection is provided to the surrounding dental tissues. This ability to remove tissue selectively with fine control especially when using a 300 m fiber makes the Nd:YAG laser an excellent instrument. There is excellent hemostasis and minimal tissue rebound when CO_2 laser is used. Indicated power setting ranges form 4–190 W depending on the nature of the tissue when used properly the pulsed layer does not create deep thermal damage resulting in much reduced post operative discomfort. Operative and post-operative bleeding with the laser is significantly less with standard instrumentation of gingivectomy and gingivoplasty. In gingivoplasty CO_2 laser are very effective. After the laser is usually used in both gingivectomy and gingivoplasty with the power setting focused and defocused mode ranging from 2 to 5 µl.

Gold and Vilardi studied the effect of Nd:YAG laser curettage on the crevicular lining of gingival tissue. They concluded that the pulsed ND:YAG laser can be used to remove the sulcular epithelium of periodontal pocket when scaling is followed by Nd:YAG laser treatment.

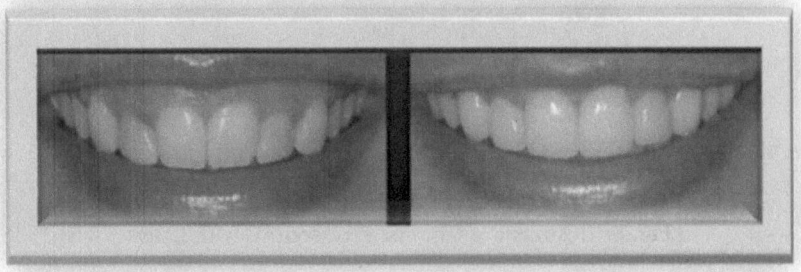

Fig. 9: Application of Lasers in Gingivectomy

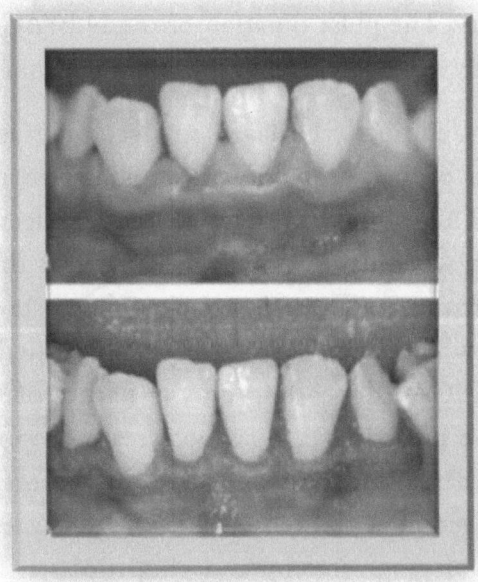

Fig. 10: Preoperative and Postoperative pictures showing the gingivectomy procedure by Lasers

Drug Induced Gingival Overgrowth

Lasers are used to treat gingival over growth. In 1998, John S. Mattsons, Richard Blankenan and Joseph J. Keene were the first to use an argon laser to remove generalized severe gingival overgrowth. Darbar and colleagues reported on the use of the CO_2 laser to treat drug-Induced gingival overgrowth. They used a combination of routine gingivectomy instruments to remove the bulk of the tissue, and then used the laser for the final contouring and coagulation. [13] [14] [15]

Patients with hyperplastic states of the gingival tissue may be treated by laser gingivectomy & no surgery is involved in these cases.

Crown Lengthening

Laser can be used very efficaciously for crown lengthening (removal of excessive gingival display) due to excessive soft tissue or a passive eruption problem. When patients have clinical crowns that appears too short and they have an uneven gingival line producing an uneven smile. Excessive tissue can be easily and quickly removed without the need for blade incision, flap reflection or suturing. Power settings are usually from 3 to 6 W of indicated power, with the beam moving from a focused to a defocused mode as necessary. To protect underlying tooth structure, a no.7 wax spatula is used in the sulcus. As lasing continues, the spatula is moved in conjunction with the laser. One must first sound the area to determine the position of the cemento-enamel junction to the crest of the tissue.

Removal of Fibromas and Papillomas

Removal of fibromas and papillomas is accomplished with minimal anaesthesia no sutures and little to no bleeding.[16] Procedure can be performed the same day preliminary impressions are made. Post-operative discomfort is tolerated with over the contour pain Medication and warm salt water rinses.[17]

Biopsies (Incisional/Excisional)

CO_2 laser is an effective instrument for soft tissue excisional biopsies with minimal intraoperative and postoperative complications and good pain control. CO_2 laser applications are suggested as an alternative method to conventional surgery on oral soft tissues.

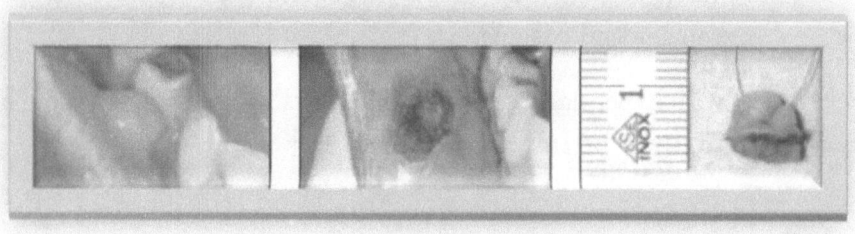

Fig. 11: Application of Lasers in Biopsy

Frenectomy

One of the most dramatic applications of the laser in periodontics is in Frenectomy. A laser frenectomy is bloodless and requires minimal anesthesia and the char layer left over the ablated frenum area allows for little/no discomfort. The operated area does not heal as quickly as a sutured wound. But the lack of post-operative pain causes delayed wound healing.[18]

This technique is particularly useful in younger patients because it is so benign compared with traditional surgery. The procedure is carried out at 4 to 5 W in the slightly defocused mode being raised as the fibre tip moved away form the attached gingiva onto the non attached tissue toward the mucosa of the vestibule. The operative time is reduced, requiring 35 seconds to 2/3 minutes.

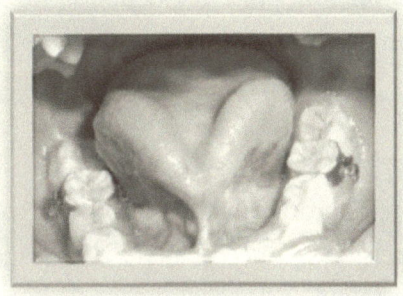
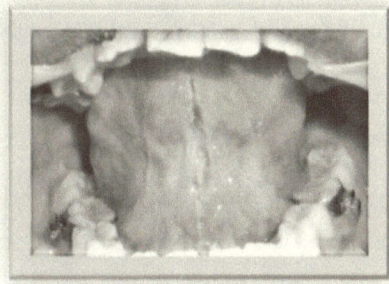

Fig. 12: Application of Lasers in Frenectomy

Vestibuloplasty

There are evidences of clinically significant improvements in vestibular depth and peri implant soft tissue situation by laser. Also, bleeding during surgery is well controlled; the patient's discomfort and pain is less than the surgery done with gingival graft. There is insufficient evidence to suggest that any specific wavelength of laser is superior to the traditional modalities of therapy. However, improved hemostasis and patient's satisfaction can be considered as advantages of adjunctive laser therapy in some clinical situations like vestibuloplasty.

Operculectomy

Operculum is nothing but the soft tissue covering the third molar that is totally or partially erupted in the oral cavity. If it is not removed, it causes pericoronitis which is the inflammation of the gingiva in relation to the crown of an incompletely erupted tooth leading to pain in the region. It can be easily removed by the Diode laser.

Gingival Depigmentation

Pigmented gingival tissue often forces patients to seek cosmetic treatment. Semiconductor diode laser light at 800 to 900nm is poorly absorbed in water, but highly absorbed in hemoglobin and other pigments. Thus, it can be readily used for gingival depigmentation procedures.

Osseous Surgery

Since laser-biologic tissue interactions are photothermal, hence, inspite of having added advantages of surgical precision, reduced collateral damage of soft tissue, reduced noise and eliminating vibrations with conventional instruments, effect of most dental lasers on bone is determinental for osseous surgery with the exeption of Er:YAG and Er,Cr:YAG. Fourier Transformation Infrared Spectra of bone surfaces has shown formation of toxic by-products that delays healing after Er:YAG laser without water coolant, and CO_2 laser irradiation. Recent clinical applicatons for Er:YAG laser in bone surgery have been reported, however, lower cutting efficiency as compared to conventional instruments and lack of depth control are its limitations.

Distal Wedge and Tuberosity Reduction

For soft tissue distal wedge and tuberosity reduction procedures, lasers offer many advantages. Common problems often associated with these procedures are the limited access for proper protocol, and the absence of keratinized tissue, especially true in the areas distal and lingual to the lower second and third molars. Furthermore, every clinician who has performed maxillary distal tuberosity reductions has faced the following scenario once the wedge is prepared and the tissue is thinned, the flaps overlap. These in turn must be further trimmed, often more than once, and often after further trimming the flaps are too short to approximate. Furthermore, these can prove to be difficult areas for access to suturing. The laser allows the operator simply vaporize or cut away the tissue as needed until the desired end result achieved. Indicated power settings range from 4 to 7W, with the beam moving from a focused to a defocused mode as needed for vaporization and fine tissue removal.

Aphthous Ulcers

One of the more remarkable laser benefits is the relief of the painful symptoms associated with aphthous ulcers. The exact mechanism by which this occurs is not known. It appears that an aphthous wound, which is painful, is converted to a laser wound, which is non painful.

The laser is set to its lowest indicated settings usually 1 to 2 W. The laser is brought into a highly defocused mode where minimal energy is being delivered to the site and then the beam is brought closer to the aphthous ulcer until the patient just begins to feel a slight sensation of discomfort or heat. At this point, using a circular motion, the aphthous ulcer is lased from its center to just beyond the erythematous halo. Slight surface alteration of the aphthous ulcer will be noted.

Herpetic Lesions

Carbon dioxide lasers have been used effectively for symptomatic relief of herpetic lesions. The results are immediate and the lesions tend to heal more quickly. The technique is exactly the same as that for the removal of aphthous ulcers. However, extreme caution should be exercised in these cases since the herpes virus may be transmitted via the laser plume.

Dentinal Hypersensitivity

Lasers have proven to be very effective in reducing or completely eliminating therapeutic sensitivity especially that due to cold.[19] The exact mechanism for the various wavelengths is not yet known. It would appear that lasers in some way effectively seal the dentinal tubules. For the CO_2 lasers, the beam is used in the lightly defocused mode and at low indicated power settings 1 to 2 W. The reported results are impressive. Meyers noted that lasing results in closure of the exposed dentinal tublues and a chance in the hydraulic conductance/rate of fluid through and lased dentine is harder than non lased deficiency the dentinal tubules and a morphologic change in the odontoblasts. [20] [21] [22]

Lasers in Oral Implantology

The gingival epithelium/biological seal becomes an important factor in implant longevity. The seal must be effective enough to prevent the ingress of bacterial plaque toxins, oral debris and other deleterious substances. The Nd:YAG laser has properties suitable for welding titanium. Carbon dioxide lasers work exceptionally well for uncovering implants whether there may be single or multiple fixtures.[23] For this indication, the CO_2 laser simply vaporizes the overlying tissue until the surgical healing is reached. This is accomplished with a defocused mode, a circular motion and indicated power setting of 3 to 6 W. This can also be referred to as a "cookie cutter" approach. The opening can then be easily contoured and enlarged as needed. When applicable, the laser eliminates the need for a flap and suturing, and reduces the level of postoperative discomfort that would normally be associated with this procedure.[24]

Laser De-Epithelialization for Enhcanced Guided Tissue Regeneration

Epithelial proliferation apically along the healing root surface has been shown to interfere with the establishment of new connective tissue attachment and underlying alveolar bone.[25]

Historically Goldman, Shapiro, Caffesse et al, Nyman et al, have tried to retard epithelial down growth. The search for a predictable method of epithelial exclusion led to the idea of applying the characteristics of laser wound periodontal therapy. This is as follows:

- The laser wound margins show thermal necrosis and formation of a firm eschear that impedes epithelial migrations.
- Decrease in wound contraction (fewer myofibroblasts) leaves a greater surface area remaining to be epithelialized.
- Reduced inflammation in the laser-induced wound may provide stimulation for epithelial migration.

- The thin layer of denatured collagen on the surface of the laser wound acts as an impervable dressing in the immediate post-operative period reducing the degree of tissue irritation from oral contents.

In this process CO_2 lasers is used to de-epithelize the gingival flaps. A more complete removal of sulcular epithelium is obtained by laser than by knives. The technique effectively removes the oral and sulcular epithelium from a gingival flap without damaging the viability of the flap during wound healing.

This concept provides a paradigm shift from the conventional use of GTR therapy and a more comprehensive therapy for treating periodontal disease with multiple lesions, concurrently in an economical manner.

Photodynamic Therapy (PDT)

Photodynamic therapy basically involves three nontoxic ingredients: visible harmless light, a nontoxic photosensitizer (i.e. a photoactivable substance) and oxygen. It is based on the principle that the photosensitizer binds to the target cells and can be activated by light of a suitable wavelength. Following activation of the photosensitizer, singlet oxygen and other reactive agents that are extremely toxic to certain cells and bacteria are produced. This singlet oxygen might cause toxic effects on the microorganisms: damage of the membrane lipids, destruction of protein and ion channels, elimination of critical metabolic enzymes, cell agglutination and inhibition of exogenous virulence factors such as lipopolysaccharide, collagenase and protease. Photosensitizers for PDT are selected for their ability to rapidly penetrate bacterial biofilms and to selectively stain and kill the prokaryotic cells under illumination while avoiding damage to human tissues.

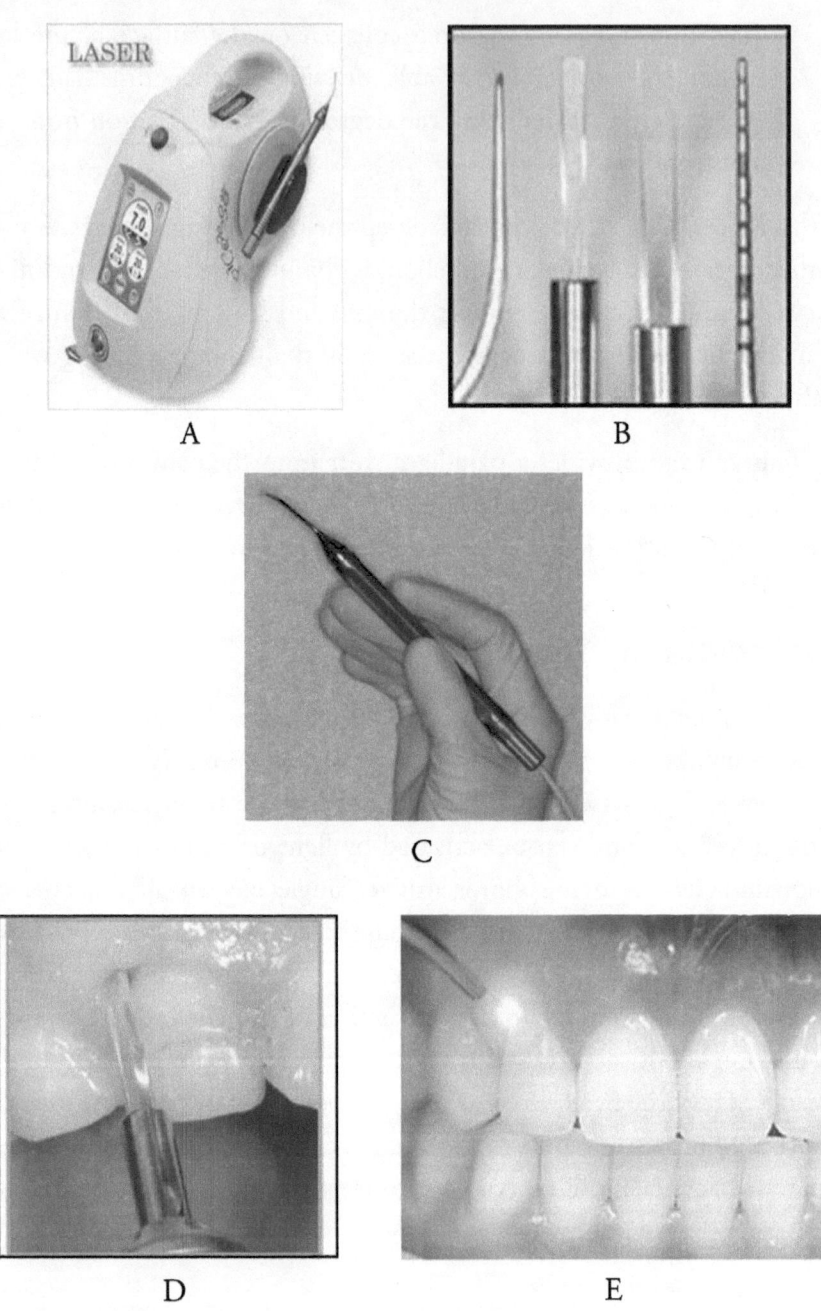

Fig. 13: A, Laser Unit. **B,** Working tips of ultrasonic scaler (left) and Er:YAG laser device (centre) with dimensions comparable to those of periodontal probe (right). **C,** Laser Handpice. **D, E,** Laser tip application on the Periodontal tissues.

Table 2: Summary of Lasers and their applications in periodontics[1]

Laser type	Wavelength (in nm)	Wave form	Delivery system	Contact	Clinical applications in periodontics
Cabondioxide (CO_2) laser	10600	Gated or continuous	Hollow waveguide/articulated arm	Beam focused at 1 to 2 mm from target surface	Soft tissue incision and ablation; subgingival curettage; biopsy; de-contamination of implant
Neodymium: Yttrium-aluminium-garnet (Nd:YAG) laser	1064	Pulsed	Flexible fiberoptic system	Surface contact required	Soft tissue incision and ablation; subgingival curettage; bacterial elimination.
Erbium: yttrium-aluminium-garnet (Er:YAG) laser	2940	Free running pulsed	Flexible fiberoptic system or Hollow waveguide	Surface contact required	Soft tissue incision and ablation; subgingival curettage; scaling; root conditioning; osteoplasty and ostectomy; degranulation and de-contamination of implants

Contd...

Laser type	Wave-length (in nm)	Wave form	Delivery system	Contact	Clinical applications in periodontics
Erbium, Chromium: yttrium-selenium-gallium-garnet (Er, Cr;YSGG) laser	2780	Free running pulsed	Air-cooled fiberoptic/ handpiece	Surface contact required	Soft tissue incision and ablation; subgingival curettage; scaling of root surfaces; osteoplasty and ostectomy
Argon (Ar) laser	488 and 514	Gated or continuous	Flexible fiberoptic system	Non-contactor contact mode	Soft tissue incision and ablation
Indium-gallium-arsenide-phosphide: Gallium-aluminium-arsenide; Gallium-arsenide InGaAsP, GaAlAs, GaAs (diode) laser	635 to 950	Gated or continuous	Flexible fiberoptic system	Surface contact required	Soft tissue incision and ablation; subgingival curettage; bacterial elimination.

APPLICATIONS OF LASERS IN ENDODONTICS

The main goals of endodontic treatment are the effective cleaning of the root-canal system. Traditional endodontic techniques use mechanical instruments, as well as ultrasound and chemical irrigation to shape, clean and completely decontaminate the endodontic system. Laser technology was introduced to endodontics with the goal of improving the results obtained with traditional procedures through the use of light energy by increasing cleaning ability and the removal of debris and the smear layer from the root canals and also improving the decontamination of the endodontic system.[26] The complexity of the root-canal system is well known. Numerous lateral canals, of various dimensions and with multiple morphologies, branch off from the principal canals. A recent study found complex anatomical structures in 75% of the teeth analyzed. The study also found residual infected pulp after the completion of chemo-mechanical preparation, both in the lateral canals and in the apical structures of vital and necrotic teeth associated with peri-radicular inflammation.[27] Laser technology was introduced to endodontics with the goal of improving the results obtained with traditional procedures through the use of light energy by increasing cleaning ability and the removal of debris and the smear layer from the root canals and also improving the decontamination of the endodontic system. Different wavelengths have been shown to be effective in significantly reducing bacteria in infected canals and studies have confirmed these results *in vitro*. Further studies have demonstrated the efficiency of lasers in combination with commonly used irrigants, such as 17% EDTA, 10% citric acid and 5.25% sodium hypochlorite.[28] The action of the chelating substances facilitates the penetration of laser light, which can penetrate into the dentinal walls up to 1mm in depth and have a stronger decontaminating effect than chemical agents. Other studies have investigated the ability of certain wavelengths to activate the irrigating solutions within the canal. This technique, which is termed laser-activated irrigation, has been shown to be statistically more effective in removing debris and the smear layer in root canals compared with traditional techniques and ultrasound.[29] A recent study by DiVito *et al.*, demonstrated that the use of the Erbium laser at sub-ablative energy density using a radial and stripped tip in combination with EDTA irrigation results in effective debris and smear layer removal without any thermal damage to the organic dentinal structure.[30] Scientific basis for the use of lasers in endodontics [31] Laser–tissue interaction the interaction of light on a target follows the rules of optical physics. Light can be reflected, absorbed, diffused or transmitted.

1. Reflection is the phenomenon of a beam of laser light hitting a target and being reflected for lack of affinity. It is therefore obligatory to wear protective eyewear to avoid accidental damage to the eyes.
2. Absorption is the phenomenon of the energy incident on tissue with affinity being absorbed and thereby exerting its biological effects.
3. Diffusion is the phenomenon of the incident light penetrating to a depth in a non-uniform manner with respect to the point of interaction, creating biological effects at a distance from the surface.
4. Transmission is the phenomenon of the laser beam being able to pass through tissue without affinity and having no effect. The interaction of laser light and tissue occurs when there is optical affinity between them. This interaction is specific and selective based on absorption and diffusion. The less affinity, the more light will be reflected or transmitted.

Effects of laser light on bacteria and dentinal walls.[32] In endodontics, lasers use the photo-thermal and photomechanical effects resulting from the interaction of different wavelengths and different parameters on the target tissues. These are dentine, the smear layer, debris, residual pulp and bacteria in all their various aggregate forms. Using different outputs, all the wavelengths destroy the cell wall due to their photo-thermal effect. Because of the structural characteristics of the different cell walls, gram-negative bacteria are more easily destroyed with less energy and radiation than gram-positive bacteria. The near infrared lasers are not absorbed by hard dentinal tissues and have no ablative effect on dentinal surfaces. The thermal effect of the radiation penetrates up to 1mm into the dentinal walls, allowing for a decontaminating effect on deeper dentine layers. The medium infrared lasers are well absorbed by the water content of the dentinal walls and consequently have a superficial ablative and decontaminating effect on the root canal surface.

Laser Wavelength Consideration[33]

The primary use of lasers in endodontics is focused on eradicating microorganisms in the root channel, especially in the lateral dentinal tubuli. This requires a wavelength that shows high transmission through hydroxyapatite and water. Absorption curves show that Nd: YAG lasers, and in particular pulsed Nd: YAG lasers, are first-choice for this application. Nd: YAG lasers show the best results in transmission and microorganism reduction measurements.

Thermal Consideration

Behrens and Gutknecht, 1993,[34] conducted in-vitro experiments on dentine slices with laser power settings that take into account even the most extreme situations, in order to determine that no thermal damage occurs in pulsed Nd: YAG laser or diode laser treatments. When measuring the root surface, a temperature of 38° C was obtained after 45-second treatment duration at 15Hz/1.5W. This value lies within the physiological area.

It must be considered that in an in-vivo situation the dental tissue is more efficiently cooled by the blood flow that surrounds the root surface.

Morphological Changes

The smear layer is completely removed and the dental tubuli are, for the most part closed through inorganic melting if the Nd: YAG laser is applied with 15Hz/1.5W settings.[35] Similar results can be expected if the 810 nm laser diode is used. If the Er: YAG laser is applied, the smear layer will be completely removed and the dental tubuli remain open.

Disinfection Effect

GUTKNECHT et al.,[36] achieved an average of 99.92% bacterial reduction in the root canal using the Nd: YAG laser with standard settings of 15 Hz at 100 mJ = 1.5 W, repeated four times for 5 to 8 sec. In 1994, Rooney et al.,[37] and Hardee et al.,[38] described reductions of 99 % when using a Nd: YAG laser in different experimental designs and bacterial combinations. Further studies examined the depth effect of the laser in the root canal dentine. In 1997, Klinke et al., were able to prove a bactericidal effect of the Nd: YAG laser at a depth of 1,000 µm. In comparison, a rinsing solution, such as NaOCl, only achieves effective bacterial reduction up to a depth of 100 µm.[39]

Clinical Procedure

The sum of all pre-clinical studies of laser-supported endodontic treatments has been the foundation for the development of a laser-supported endodontic therapeutic plan. Based on their specific bactericidal effect, laser procedures have been integrated in the conventional endodontic therapeutic concept to indisputably improve conventional therapy. Clinical studies have led to the further establishment of a laser supported therapeutic plan and have allowed results to be verified over defined periods of time in order to enable statements to be made about the success prospects of laser-supported endodontic treatments.[40] Indications and contra-indications for laser supported endodontic treatments[41] Laser-supported treatments should be favored when treating patients that show one or several of the following symptoms:

1. Teeth with a purulent pulpitis or pulp necrosis
2. Teeth, of which the crown and root pulp show gangrenous changes
3. Teeth with peri-apical lesions (peri-apical gap from 1 mm, up to granulomas with a diameter of 5 mm and more)
4. Teeth with a peri-apical abscess
5. Teeth with lateral canals that lead to periodontal involvement
6. Absorption of the apex caused by inflammation or trauma
7. Teeth that have been treated for at least three months without success (with alternating rinsing and medicinal inlay

Diagnosis of Pulp Vitality by Laser[42]

A Laser Doppler flowmetry was developed by Tenland in 1982 and later by Hollway in 1983. This method uses Helium-Neon and diode lasers at a lower power of 1 or 2 mw. Laser Doppler flowmetry is a noninvasive method of assessing and accurately measuring the rate of blood flow in a tissue. The pulp is a highly vascular tissue and cardiac blood flow in the supplying artery is transmitted through pulsations. These pulsations are apparent on the laser doppler monitor of vital teeth and absent in the non-vital teeth. The blood flux level is much higher in vital than non- vital teeth. Currently, the vitality can be interpreted from a signal on the screen. Differential diagnosis of pulpitis can be done by laser stimulation.[42]

a) Normal Pulp and acute Pulpitis

When normal pulp is stimulated by the pulsed Nd: YAG laser at 2W and 20 pulses per second (pps) at a distance approximately 10 mm from the tooth surface, pain is produced within 20 to 30 seconds and disappears a couple of seconds after the laser stimulation is stopped. In the case of acute pulpitis the pain is induced immediately after laser application and continues for more than 30 seconds after stopping the laser stimulation.

b) Acute Serous Pulpitis and Acute Suppurative Pulpitis

Differential diagnosis of acute serous pulpitis and acute suppurative pulpitis can be obtained by combining the measurement of electric current resistance of caries and the pain duration induced by laser stimulation. If the electric current resistance is greater than 15.1 m^2 and the patient experiences continuous pain for more than 30 seconds, the diagnosis is acute serous pulpitis. When the value of resistance is less than 15.0 m^2 and there is continuous pain for more than 30 seconds, the diagnosis is acute suppurative pulpitis. Caries impedence of less than 15.0 m^2 indicates that no hard healthy dentin exists between the caries and the pulp chamber.

Lasers in Pulp Capping[42]

Accessory treatment by laser for Indirect Pulp-capping Pulsed Nd: YAG laser is used and black ink applied on the tooth surface. Air spray cooling is needed to prevent pulp damage resulting from the laser energy provided by 2W and 20pps for less than 1 second to the area. CO laser can also be used. In some cases, it is recommended that this laser be used with 38% silver ammonium solution. These treatments should be performed under local anesthesia.

Direct Pulp Capping by Laser[42]

CO_2 laser irradiation is performed at 1 or 2W after irrigating with 8% sodium hypochlorite and 3% hydrogen peroxide for more than 5 minutes. Calcium hydroxide paste must be used to dress the exposed pulp after laser treatment, after which the cavity should be tightly sealed with cement such as polycarboxylate cement. Pulsed Nd: YAG, argon, semiconductor diode, and Er: YAG can also be used.

Laser Ablation and Accessory Treatment for Vital Pulp Amputation[42]

The lasers used are CO_2, pulsed Nd: YAG, He, and low power semiconductor diode lasers and middle power semiconductor diode lasers. The usage of CO_2 laser is time consuming and pulp tissue may be damaged due to several exposures. Pulsed Nd: YAG causes damage to the pulp tissue and thereby showed a low success rates so it should be used only for pulp hemostasis, sedation, anti-inflammatory effects, and stimulation of remaining pulpal cells.

Laser in Analgesia

Certain wavelengths of laser energy interfere with the sodium pump mechanism, change cell membrane permeability, alter temporarily the endings of sensory neurons, and block depolarization of C and A fibers of the nerves. In this area the pulsed â Nd: YAG laser has commanded the most attention. The use of lasers in endodontic therapy has been extensively studied for the past 15 years and proven to have many advantages over conventional methods. Results suggest that the laser is an effective tool for removal of debris, the smear layer and obturation materials, as well as being an effective is infection tool.

Laser in Apicoectomy, Retrograde and Endodontic Apical Cavity Preparation, and Periapical Curettage

Advantages of laser over scalpel are greater precision, a relatively bloodless and post-surgical course, sterile surgical area, minimal swelling and scarring, coagulation, vaporization and cutting, minimal or no suturing and much less or no post surgical pain.[43] Permeability of dentin exposed by apicoectomy is one of the causes of endodontic surgery failure because micro-leakage and bacterial contamination trigger inflammation. The use of lasers resulted in smoother surfaces and more homogenous dentin fusion and recrystallization, which occluded[44] tubules and decreased permeability. Apicoectomy with burs and treatment of apical surface with Nd: YAG laser; Apicoectomy with bur, root end cavity preparation with ultrasound, filling with MTA; treatment of apical surface with CO_2 laser and apicoectomy with Er: YAG laser and treatment of apical surface with Nd: YAG laser.[45]

Laser Treatment of Periapical Lesions of Sinus Tract

Laser therapy is recommended for cases for which apicoectomy or periapical curettage cannot be performed, or for which standard endodontic treatment cannot be performed, because of deep post in the root canal. This treatment can be performed to accelerate wound healing in combination with endodontic or surgical treatment. Pulsed Nd: YAG and CO_2 lasers are recommended for these treatments.[43]

APPLICATIONS OF LASERS IN ORAL MEDICINE

Oromucosal Pathologies

Leukoplakia

It is defined by WHO as 'a white patch or plaque that cannot be characterized clinically or pathologically as any other disease.' It is considered as a common precancerous lesion of the oral mucosa. There are different kinds of treatment for this lesion including scalpel excision, electro cautery, cryosurgery, laser surgery and medications. The lesions can be removed with laser and encourages regeneration of new, healthy epithelium. Small lesions can be removed with a carbon dioxide laser with a margin of 3 to 4 mm. The decision of whether excision or vaporization should be done is based on the texture and thickness of the lesion. Thickened hyper keratotic lesions have less water content, therefore, vaporization cannot be done. Diffuse lesions cannot be managed by excision. In such lesions, carbon dioxide lasers can be used in a defocused mode to produce cross hatched pattern. The disadvantage of vaporization is that, a specimen cannot be taken and sent for pathological examination, so, the histology of the lesion cannot be determined.[46]

Oral Lichen Planus

It is a chronic inflammatory disease that causes bilateral white striations, papules, or plaques on buccal mucosa, tongue and gingiva. The oral lesions are exhibited in two forms: reticular and erosive. The reticular form is characterized by interlacing white lines called Wickham's striae. The erosive form appears as erythematous area with central ulceration. Erosive lichen planus can be controlled by laser treatment. Carbon dioxide laser should be used along with selected local and systemic medications. The contact Nd: YAG laser with round probe can also be used.[47]

Oral Sub-Mucous Fibrosis

Oral sub-mucous fibrosis (OSMF) is a chronic disease characterized by progressive inability to open the mouth. Various treatment modalities are available for its management, but these have largely been ineffective. In the modern era, the use of laser to release fibrotic bands leads to healing with minimal scarring, thereby decreasing the probability of procedure induced trismus. Diode laser is a portable device which delivers rays through a fiber-optic cable and, hence, can be delivered to relatively 'difficult-to-access' areas. Its cutting depth is less than 0.01 mm, and thus preserves tissues beyond this depth. It gives a precise line of controlled cutting without damaging the muscles and deeper structures. Hence, laser therapy eliminates the use of grafts, to close the defect in spite of extensive resection. It yields excellent functional results.[48]

Herpes Simplex Virus Infections

Herpes simplex virus types 1 and 2 are the main infectious agents associated with oral and genital ulcerations. Different methods of HSV identification and treatment of oral cavity lesions are available, including the use of oral, intravenous or topical antiviral medications. Low-level laser therapy (LLLT) can be used in association with conventional therapy. The choice of treatment method will depend on the number, location and size of the lesions.[49] LLLT presents both anti-inflammatory and analgesic effects, contributing to tissue repair and fibroblast proliferation and an increase in the interval between infections; moreover, it does not contribute in viral resistance.

Recurrent Aphthous Ulcers

It is the most common oral ulcerative lesion. The exact cause of these ulcers is unknown. Recently, LLLT has been used as the treatment modality. It helps in immediate pain relief and accelerates wound healing. According to De Souza et al, there is a significant pain relief in the same session after laser treatment and the lesion is totally regressed in 4 days. When steroids are used, it takes 5 to 7 days for regression.[50]

Walsh LJ has done a tremendous amount of research on the proposed mechanisms of the action of LLLT on both hard and soft tissues and has proposed that cold lasers (LLLT lasers) accelerate wound healing and reduce pain by perhaps 'stimulating oxidative phosphorylation in mitochondria and modulating inflammatory responses.'[51, 52]

Orofacial Pain

Trigeminal Neuralgic Pain

Trigeminal neuralgia is a neuropathic disorder of the trigeminal nerve that causes episodes of intense pain in the eyes, lips, nose, scalp, forehead, and jaw, with the majority of cases being unilateral (>95%).[53] This lancinating pain is typically in the distribution of the second and third divisions of the trigeminal nerve and can be triggered by facial movement, cold temperature, talking, and other common activities.[54] According to Eckerdal and Bastin, low-level laser of 830 nm wavelength was efficient in the treatment of 81% of patients, with 42% of them having no pain after a year.[55] In contrast, there was an improvement in 50% of patients who had been treated with injection of alcohol and only 20% remained pain-free after a year. It has also been shown that com pared to placebo, low-level laser is significantly effective in pain relief.[56]

Myofacial Pain

Myofacial pain dysfunction syndrome (MPDS) is the most common reason for pain and limited function of the masticatory system. The effects of LLLs for controlling the discomfort of patients are investigated frequently. Several studies have shown that use of 830 nm wave length laser in several appointments can reduce or eliminate myofacial pain.[57, 58] Shirani et al evaluated the efficacy of a LLLT producing 660 and 890 nm wavelengths and concluded LLLT was an effective treatment for pain reduction in MPDS patients.[59]

Temporomandibular Joint Disorder Pain

Temporomandibular joint (TMJ) pain is recognized as an important source of disability that leads to considerable socioeconomic costs as a result of medical treatments, surgical interventions, and frequent absences from work.[60, 61] A potential noninvasive treatment for TMJ pain is LLLT. The relative clinical efficacy of LLLT for the treatment of temporomandibular disorders (TMD) is controversial. Some authors reported the efficacy of LLLT to be superior to placebo therapy.[62] While others found no significant differences between LLLT and placebo for measures of TMJ pain.[63]

Mucositis Pain

Pathologic evaluation of mucositis reveals mucosal thinning leading to a shallow ulcer thought to be caused by inflammation and depletion of the epithelial basal layer with subsequent denudation and bacterial infection.

'Low' or 'low and middle' energy (output power ranged from 5 to 200 mw) irradiation with helium/neon laser (wavelength 632.8 nm) has been reported to be a simple atraumatic technique (with no known toxicity in clinical setting), useful in the treatment of mucositis of various origins.

Salivary Gland Pathologies

Sialolithiasis

Sialolithiasis is the most common disease of the salivary glands. It is characterized by the development of calcifications (sialoliths) that accumulate within the salivary gland parenchyma and associated ductal systems. Most of the sialoliths are found in the sub-mandibular gland.[64] Various types of lasers have been employed to treat sialolithiasis, including carbon dioxide, diode, Ho: Yag and Nd: YAG lasers. Among these diode laser has been reported to have more advantages. It has a greater absorption by hemoglobin, oxy-hemoglobin and melanin, thereby making its penetration depth smaller than Nd-YAG laser. Owing to the smaller penetration in blood rich tissues diode laser is accepted to be safe in the adjacent tissues.[65] Due to its excellent cutting and coagulation ability, diode laser is an alternative option for the soft-tissue surgery.

Mucocele

Mucocele is a common lesion of the oral mucosa that results from an alteration of minor salivary glands due to a mucous accumulation. Mucocele involves mucin accumulation causing limited swelling. CO_2 laser has a high water absorption rate and is well absorbed by all soft tissues with high water content. In addition its effects on adjacent tissues are minimal. These properties make CO_2 laser the perfect surgical treatment for oral soft tissues.[66] The cut is precise and does not affect the muscle layer, causes minimal hemorrhage and almost no acute inflammatory reaction. The operation time is short (3 to 5 minutes) making it a convenient treatment for children and patients who cannot withstand long treatment.[67]

Biopsy

With regard to the technique used, we can distinguish biopsy as incisional and excisional. The excisional biopsy is the removal of the lesion in total, allowing, at the same time, to carry both a diagnostic and therapeutic procedure. The incisional biopsy involves the removal of one or more fragments representative of the lesion, together with the adjacent tissues, deep and surrounding it, and only after the histological examination, it is possible to establish the treatment of residual lesion.[68] It is possible to make withdrawals of histological samples using two different procedures, which is used respectively, the scalpel and the laser. The laser biopsies present some advantages compared those made with the scalpel: generally these interventions do not require anesthesia or sutures and the healing of the donor site, at least in the initial stages, it is more rapid. The laser most commonly used for this purpose are the diode laser, KTP laser, CO_2 laser, Nd: YAG laser, Er: YAG laser.[69]

APPLICATIONS OF LASERS IN ORTHODONTICS

Lasers in Orthodontics-Clinical Applications

Lasers in Etching

Application of laser energy to an enamel surface causes localized melting and ablation and therefore removal of enamel.[70] Enamel removal (etching), results primarily from the micro explosion of entrapped water in the enamel, in addition there may be some melting of the hydroxyl-apatite crystals. Laser irradiation, in particular, causes thermally induced changes on the enamel surface. It causes surface roughening and irregularity similar to that of acid-etching to a depth of 10-20 μm, depending on the type of laser and the energy applied to the surface.[71] von Fraunhoufer et al. studied the effectiveness of a commercial Nd: YAG laser in etching dental enamel for direct bonding of orthodontic appliances. If shear bond strength of 0.60 kg/mm is taken as the minimum acceptable value for clinical use, the findings of the study indicate that laser etching must be performed at the maximum power output of the American Dental Nd: YAG laser to achieve consistent surface conditioning.

Laser for De-Bonding Procedure

Lasers have been tried in both acid etching and de-bonding of brackets with promising results. This approach has been shown to be efficient for de-bonding, resulting in a decreased adhesive remnant index and a relatively small increase in pulp temperature. In particular, application of Nd: YAG and CO_2 lasers have shown satisfying results and minimal side-effects from the increase in pulp temperature. Strob et al.[72] studied on the efficiency of using CO_2 and Nd: YAG lasers in de-bonding ceramic brackets from the enamel surface. Laser-aided de-bonding technique was found to significantly reduce the residual de-bonding force, the risk of enamel damage and the incidence of failure as compared with the conventional de-bonding techniques. Therefore, this method has the potential to be more a-traumatic (less painful) and safer (less risk of enamel damage) for the patient.

Light Curing Lasers

The extended placement time offered by light-cured adhesives allows more accurate bracket positioning. The major disadvantage of these adhesives has been the 20–40 s required to set each bracket with a curing light. Although the shear bond strength of light-cured adhesives is comparable to that of chemically activated adhesives, it increases dramatically between 5 min and 24 h after placement, with the bond strength at 5 min only 60-70% of the bond strength at 24 h could be achieved. BisGMA, the most common monomer in composite adhesives, is polymerized when one of the double bonds at either end of the polymer is broken and then attached to another BisGMA polymer. Recent research has focused on the argon laser's ability to achieve photo polymerization of composite resins. Photo activated dental resins use a dike tone initiator such as camphoroquinone and a reducing agent such as a tertiary amine to initiate polymerization. This photo-initiator system is very sensitive to light in the blue region of the visible light spectrum, with a peak of activity centered around 480 nm. The argon laser is monochromatic and emits light over a narrow band of wavelengths in the blue, green spectrum (457.9-514.5 nm), making it ideally suited to polymerize composite. Talbot et al.[73] determined whether argon laser irradiation of enamel has concluded that argon lasers can be used to bond orthodontic brackets, achieving bond strengths similar to those attained with conventional light curing resins.

Using lasers for orthodontic treatment management and enhancing aesthetics

Orthodontic patients are interested in more than just "straight teeth." They are interested in well-aligned, beautiful white teeth; ideal function and occlusion; ideal gingival esthetics; well-proportioned faces and gorgeous smiles. Furthermore, patients would like this to be accomplished in a reasonable amount of time. Recently, the Soft-tissue laser has gained attention as an effective tool to help manage treatment and enhance the esthetic outcomes.

Lasers in Orthodontics-Non Clinical Applications

Laser Scanning

Laser scanners are capable of producing detailed models;[74] however, the scanning process requires the subject to remain still for a period of seconds to a minute or more while the scanner revolves around the subjects head, because the laser provides only the surface map and cannot provide color information for the texture map. A color camera that is registered with the laser scanner provides this information. In studies of laser scanning of plastic and plaster mannequin heads, investigators reported a 0.6 mm variance of localization in the three axes (x, y and z) when using pre-labeled anthropometric land marks. Three-dimensional computerized data from a laser scanner can also be transformed using computer aided manufacturing and stereo-lithography techniques to produce orthodontic appliances such as splints, computerized wire bending, e-models, and surgical simulation models. The self-corrected mechanism of the laser scanner in adjusting for image distortion gives flexibility for clinical research. The software can be used to merge images taken from different perspectives, thus eliminating undercuts. Studies involving dental casts can be performed with ease because computerized 3D wire-frame diagrams allow models to be cut, superimposed, and measured in the computer. Measuring changes in area and length of curvatures gives more insight for many data sets (figure 14a).

For craniofacial anomalies, various studies could be performed regarding cleft lip repair, asymmetrical facial growth, change of head shape, and nasal molding procedures (figure 14b). It was found in all cases that the scanner produced more accurate measurements in height (x) and width (y) but less accurate measurements in depth (z). For inter-molar width, the scanner tended to produce smaller values than the manual measurement, but it produced larger values when measuring palatal depth (figure 14c).

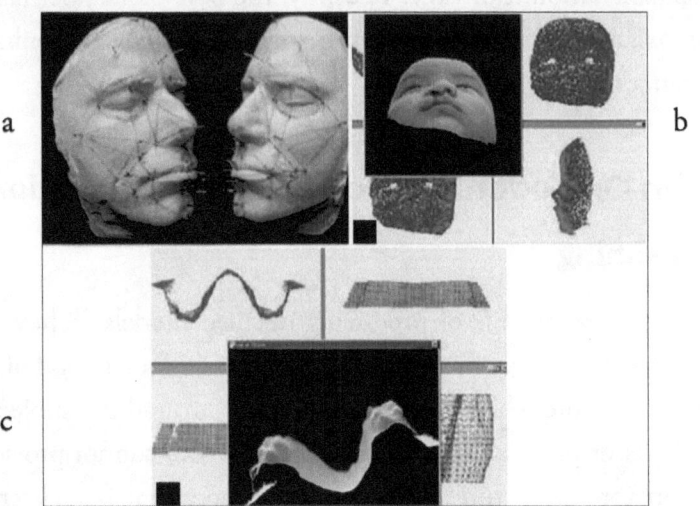

Figure 14: (a) Laser scanning producing detailed models, e-models, and surgical simulation model. (b) Laser scanning can be used to produce details about the craniofacial abnormalities, their exact location and three dimensional details. (c) Measurement of palatal depth using laser scanning

Laser Holography

A new tool for measuring tooth movement-laser holography offers an accurate, non invasive approach for determining movement in 3 dimensions. The stresses generated in the periodontal ligament when the crown of a tooth is subjected to a force have important ramifications for the study of orthodontic tooth movement and periodontal disease. In particular, the orthodontist desires to relate the force system applied to the teeth to the center of rotation and the magnitude of tooth displacement.

Previously, tooth displacements have been studied from a number of approaches: (1) Analytical models, (2) physical models, and (3) direct measurement *in vivo*.

The effects of force on the supporting periodontium and, in turn, tooth movement have also been studied by constructing physical models in photo-elastic plastic and analyzing photo-elastically the stress distribution produced by the applied force. Unfortunately, the attempts at mathematical modeling by an analytical approach as well as photo-elastic techniques have been limited by a number of oversimplifying assumptions, such as (1) the anatomy of the root, periodontal ligament, and alveolar bone were represented by idealized geometric forms, (2) the physical characteristics of the supporting structures were assumed to be homogeneous, isotropic, and linear, whereas the structures of interest here are non-homogeneous, anisotropic, and nonlinear. Furthermore, in most instances the model was two-dimensional.

Laser Welding

The joining of the metal framework is frequently necessary to create individual orthodontic appliances and to achieve efficient treatment procedures. Recent method employed for joining metal frameworks is laser welding to weld dental alloys, crystals of YAG, with added neodymium are mainly used to emit laser beams. The advantages of laser-welding are-no solder, and thus no corrosion at the joint, small focus and an argon shielding atmosphere prevents the oxidation around the welding zone.

Laser Specular Reflectance

The non-invasive technique, laser specular reflectance, also uses a preselected area of the wire surface. The three-dimensional structure of this area determines the diffuse scattered part of the laser light impinging on the surface and thus the structure of the whole region is used to calculate the roughness of the wire. The drawbacks of the method are an exacting adjustment and the limitation to rough nesses smaller than the wavelength of the laser light used. It is impossible to identify a surface roughness that is beyond this limit and all doubtful cases have to be examined against another method.

Various Adjunctive Procedures in Orthodontic Treatment

Creating Access for Bracket Placement

The diode laser can be used to remove tissue (gingivectomy and gingivoplasty) and provide access for bracket/band/button attachment. These procedures provide earlier attachment to teeth and can significantly reduce treatment times. Usually, cuspids are the last teeth bonded due to their slow eruption, delayed passive eruption or impaction. The diode laser can be used to assist the clinician in avoiding these situations by directly attaching the bracket or placing a band.

Establishing Tooth Proportionality

Most clinicians position the brackets (directly or indirectly) either by measuring a prescribed distance from the incisal edge or visualizing and positioning the bracket in the center of the clinical crown. Both methods are acceptable and have performed adequately for many years. Problems with these bracket-positioning methods tend to arise when the clinical crown is not equal to the anatomic crown in length, a common finding in adolescent orthodontic patients. Measurement from the incisal edge may result in an acceptable occlusal outcome but may result in poor oral hygiene due to encroachment of the bracket on the gingival margin. Bracket position in the center of the clinical crown would be too incisal, resulting in unwanted incisor intrusion and reduction of the incisal display at rest and on smile. The diode laser can be used at the initial placement visit, prior to positioning the bracket, to improve the proportionality and allow the position of the central incisors to be maintained during smile.

Oral Hygiene

Chronic poor oral hygiene in orthodontic patients results in gingival overgrowth, pseudo-pocket formation, and plaque-retention problems, usually resulting in increased treatment times, unsatisfactory patients and parents, and ultimately a less-than-desirable esthetic result. These problems are difficult to overcome by the patient alone, and are rarely resolved completely by using the traditional methods. The diode laser can be used to remove the pseudo-pockets, providing access for patients to improve their oral hygiene and also provide better access for topical fluoride application. This procedure can often be combined with gingival contouring for improved gingival aesthetics, and can be performed at any point during treatment or at the de-bonding visit itself.

Apthous Ulcer Management

The diode laser can be used in noncontact mode (1-2 mm away from the tissue) to irradiate the ulcer for approximately 30 s. In our experience, the patient reports an immediate reduction of pain. The procedure creates a non-painful laser wound that replaces the painful ulceration.

Gingival Contouring and Shaping

Gingival shape refers to the 2D curvature of the gingival margin. Gingival-shape problems include gingival margin discrepancies and improper zenith (apex of the curvature of the gingival-margin for a given tooth) locations. Gingival contour refers to the 3D architecture of the gingiva characterized by sharp interdental papillae and tapered gingival margins. Gingival-contour problems include rolled margins and inflamed papillae.

Assessing Patient Pain During Dental Laser Treatment[75, 76]

Low-level laser therapy (LLLT) has been shown by many investigators to produce analgesic effects in various therapeutic and clinical applications. Laser analgesia is a new treatment modality and has the advantages of being non-invasive, easy to administer, and having no known adverse tissue reactions. It is worthwhile to look into its potential applications in orthodontics.

Many researchers have reported that Nd: YAG,[77] He-Ne,[72] and Ga-Al-As diode lasers[78-80] have analgesic effects for reducing orthodontic pain. Moreover, local CO_2 laser therapy has been found effective in reducing the pain associated with orthodontic force applications.[80] Lim *et al*.[76] concluded that LLLT effectively controls pain caused by the application of the first arch wire, but it does not affect the start of pain after the first arch wire is placed and does not alter the most painful day. According to findings, LLLT reduces the prevalence of pain after multi-banding compared to a control group at 6 and 30 h.[79] On the other hand, some studies in the literature have shown that LLLT offers no significant pain reduction after separation or placement of arch-wires.[78-82] In conclusion, induction of laser analgesia is a new treatment modality that has the advantages of being non-invasive, being easy to apply and to have no known adverse tissue reactions.

APPLICATIONS OF LASERS IN PROSTHODONTICS

1. Fixed prosthesis/esthetics

A. Crown lengthening: Clinical scenarios where crown lengthening methods are specified within esthetic zone need attention to attain esthetic results. Crown lengthening methods with the help of lasers are included in following situation:

1. Caries at gingival margin
2. Cuspal fracture extending apically to the gingival margin
3. Endodontic perforations near the alveolar crest.
4. Insufficient clinical crown length.
5. Difficulty in a placement of finish line coronal to the biological width.
6. Need to develop a ferrule.
7. Unaesthetic gingival architecture.
8. Cosmetic enhancements.

Lasers offer unparallel accuracy and operator control and may be helpful for finely tracing incision lines and shaping the desired gingival margin outline. All the other crown lengthening methods has disadvantages in surgical approach healing time is longer, post healing gingival margin position is doubtful and patient compliance is poor as it needs use of anesthesia and scalpel for electro-surgery, the heat liberated has effect on pulp and bone leading to pulp death or bone necrosis.[17]

B. Soft tissue management around abutments: Argon laser energy has peak absorption in hemoglobin, thus, providing excellent hemostasis and well regulated coagulation and vaporization of oral tissues. These characteristics are beneficial for retraction and hemostasis of the gingival tissue in preparation for an impression during a crown and bridge method. Argon laser with 300 um fiber, and a power setting of 1.0W, continuous wave delivery, and the fiber is placed into the sulcus in contact with the tissue. In a sweeping motion, the fiber is moved around the tooth. It is dominant to contact the fiber tip with the bleeding vessels. Provide suction and water spray in the field. Gingivoplasty may also be done using argon laser.

C. Modification of soft tissue around laminates: The removal and re-contouring of gingival tissues cover can be easily efficient with the argon laser. The laser can be used as a primary surgical instrument to detach excessive gingival tissue, whether diseased, secondary to drug therapy or orthodontic treatment. The laser will detach tissue and supply hemostasis and tissues join the wound.

D. Osseous crown lengthening: Like teeth mineralized matrix of bone contains mainly of hydroxyapatite. The water content and hydroxyapatite produce for the high absorption of the Er: YAG laser light in the bone. Er: YAG laser has potential for bone ablation.

E. Formation of ovate pontic sites: There are many causes of the inappropriate pontic site. Two of the most common causes are inadequate compression of alveolar plates after an extraction and non-replacement of a fractured alveolar plate. Inappropriate pontic site results in unesthetic and non-self-cleansing pontic design. For favorable pontic design re-contouring of soft and bony tissue may be required. Soft tissue surgery may achieve with the soft tissue lasers and osseous surgery may achieve with erbium family of lasers. The use of an ovate pontic receptor site is of great value when trying to produce a natural maxillary anterior fixed bridge. This is easily good with the use of a laser.

F. Altered passive eruption management: Lasers can be easily to control passive eruption problems. When the patients have clinical crowns that appear too short or when they have a jagged gingival line creating an uneven smile, excessive tissue can be detached without the need for blade incisions, flap reflection, or suturing.[83]

G. Laser troughing: Lasers can be used to produce a groove around a tooth before impression taking. This can be restored for retraction cord, electrocautery, and the use of hemostatic agents. The results are obvious, well regulated, minimize impingement of epithelial attachment, cause less bleeding during the impression, decrease postoperative problems and chair time.[4] It changes the biological width of the gingiva. After laser grooving, the impression is taken and sent to the lab for prosthetic work. The main function of the marginal finish line is to keep the biological width, it acts as the termination point of tooth preparation, help in ease of fabrication, helps in taking a proper impression. In brittle teeth to keep the biological width and finish line laser grooving plays a main role.[84]

H. Bleaching: Esthetics and smile are main situation in our modern society. Bleaching of teeth can be achieved in the Dental OPD. Diode lasers are used to bleach teeth without causing much tooth sensitivity and modification of the complexion of the tooth.

I. Removal of veneer: Restoration can be removed without cutting with the help of laser beams. The laser energy passes through porcelain glass unchanged and is occupied by the water molecules present in the adhesive. Debonding takes place at the junction of the silane and the resin without causing any trauma to the underlying tooth.

J. Crown fractures at the gingival margins: Er: YAG or Er, Cr: YSGG lasers can be moved out to permit correct exposure of the fracture margin. [85]

2. Implantology

Dental lasers are used for methods in implantology such as implant recovery, implant site preparation and detach of diseased tissue around the implant.

A. Implant recovery: Thus, the placement of implant and its combination into the osseous substrate, the method of treatment is surgically exposing the implant, wait for the tissue to heal and start with impressions and fabrication of the restoration. Use of lasers can proceed this method because the implant can be exposed, and impressions can be obtained at the same appointment. All types of lasers can be used to release dental implants. There is minimal tissue shrinkage after laser surgery, which tells that the tissue margins will continue at the same level after healing.[86, 87] In addition, the use of laser can detach the trauma to the tissues of flap reflection and suture placement.

B. Implant site preparation: Lasers can be used for the placement of mini implants generally in patients with potential bleeding problems, to give bloodless surgery in the bone.

C. Removal of diseased tissue around the implant: Lasers can be used to restore implants by sterilizing their surfaces with laser energy. Diode, CO_2 & Er: YAG lasers can be used for this reason. Lasers can be used to remove granulation tissue in case there is inflammation around an Osseointegrated implant.[87, 88]

3. Removable Prosthetics

The creation of removable full and partial dentures depend on the preoperative analysis of the supporting hard and soft tissue structures and their proper preparation.[83] Lasers may now be used to perform most pre-prosthetic surgeries. These methods involve hard and soft tissue tuberosity reduction, torus removal, and treatment of inappropriate residual ridges involving undercut and irregularly resorbed ridges, treatment of unsupported soft tissues, and hard and soft tissue malformation. Lasers may be used to treat the problem of hyperplastic tissue and nicotinic stomatitis under the palate of a full or partial denture and ease the irritation of epulis, denture stomatitis, and other problems related with long term wear of ill-fitting dentures. Stability, retention, function, and esthetics of removable prostheses may be increased by proper laser manipulation of the soft tissues and underlying osseous structure.

A. Treatment of unsuitable alveolar ridges: Alveolar resorption is uniform in vertical and lateral dimensions. Thus, irregular resorption occurs in one of the dimensions, making an inappropriate ridge. As the available denture, bearing area is decreased, the load on the remaining tissue increases, which leads to an ill-fitting prosthesis, with irritation. To detach sharp bony projections and to smooth the residual ridge soft tissue lasers surgery to uncover the bone may be produced with any number of soft tissue wavelengths (CO_2, diode, Nd: YAG,) Hard tissue surgery may be produced with the erbium family of wavelengths

B. Treatment of undercut alveolar ridges: There are many reasons of undercut alveolar ridges. Two of the most common reasons are dilated tooth sockets that result from inadequate compression of the alveolar plates after an extraction and non-replacement of a fractured alveolar plate. Naturally, occurring undercuts such as those found in the lower anterior alveolus or where a prominent pre-maxilla is present may be a reason of soft tissue trauma, ulceration, and pain when prosthesis is moved on such a ridge. Soft tissue surgery may be produced with any of the soft tissue lasers. Osseous surgery may be produced with the erbium family of lasers. Common surgery includes of detaching wedges of soft tissue from the alveolar crest until the wound edges are closed. Any of the soft tissue lasers are able to produce this method.[89, 90]

C. Treatment of enlarged tuberosity: The most common cause for enlarged tuberosity usually is soft tissue hyperplasia and alveolar hyperplasia lead the over- eruption of unopposed maxillary molar teeth. The expand tuberosity may stop the posterior extension of the upper and lower dentures, thereby, decreasing their planning for mastication and their strength. The bulk of the hyperplastic tuberosity may rest toward the palate. The soft tissue decrease may be accomplished with any of the soft tissue lasers.

D. Surgical treatment of tori and exostoses: Prosthetic problems may arise if maxillary tori or exostoses are large or irregular in shape. Tori and exostoses are formed mainly of compact bone. They may cause ulceration of oral mucosa. These bony protuberances also may interfere with lingual bars or flanges of mandibular prostheses. Soft tissue lasers may be use to expose the exostoses and erbium lasers may be use for the osseous reduction.[91]

E. Soft tissue lesions: Persistent trauma from a sharp denture flange or over compression of the posterior dam area may produce a fibrous tissue response. Hyper plastic fibrous tissue may be formed at the junction of the hard and soft palate as a reaction to constant trauma and irritation from the posterior dam area of the denture. The lesion may be excised with any of the soft tissue lasers and the tissue allowed re-epithelialized.

RECENT ADVANCES IN LASERS

Waterlase system is a revolutionary dental device that uses laser energised water to cut or ablate soft and hard tissue and provide periodontists with the opportunity to perform more procedures in fewer appointments with less need for anesthesia, scalpels and drill.[1]

Periowave, a photodynamic disinfection system utilises nontoxic dye (photosensitizer) in combination with a low-intensity lasers enabling singlet oxygen molecules to destroy bacteria. After applying light-sensitive drug (photosensitizer), low-intensity laser is directed on the area treated with the drug resulting in phototoxic reactions. Although the use of photosensitizers for complete suppression of the anaerobic perio-pathogens have been suggested, however, the same is not true for facultative anaerobes.[1]

HAZARDS OF LASERS

Eye Hazards

The potential for injury to the different structures of the eye depends upon which structure absorbs the energy. Laser radiation may damage the cornea, lens or retina depending on the wavelength, intensity of the radiation and the absorption characteristics of different eye tissues.

Ocular Image

Wavelengths between 400 nm and 1400 nm are transmitted through the curved cornea and lens and focused on the retina. Intra beam viewing of a point source of light (Fig. 15) produces a very small spot on the retina resulting in a greatly increased power density and an increased chance of damage. A large source of light such as a diffuse reflection of a laser beam produces light that enters the eye at a large angle called an extended source. An extended source produces a relatively large image on the retina (Fig. 14) and energy is not concentrated on a small area on the retina as in a point source.[2]

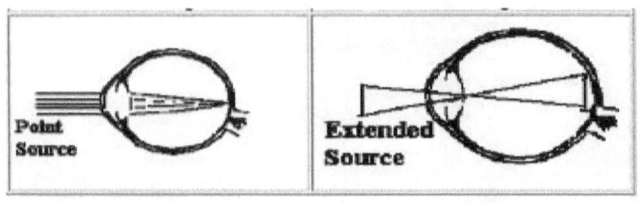

Fig: 15: Point source and extended source making an image on the retina

Effects of Irradiation on Eyes

Ultraviolet-B+C (100–315 nm)

The surface of the cornea absorbs all UV of these wavelengths which produce a photokeratitis (welders flash) by a photochemical process which cause a denaturation of proteins in the cornea. This is a temporary condition because the corneal tissues regenerate very quickly.

Ultraviolet-A (315–400 nm)

The cornea, lens and aqueous humour allow Ultraviolet radiations of these wavelengths and the principal absorber is the lens. Photochemical processes denature proteins in the lens resulting in the formation of cataracts.[2]

Visible light and Infrared-A (400–1400 nm)

The cornea, lens and vitreous fluid are transparent to electromagnetic radiation of these wavelengths. Damage to the retinal tissue occurs by absorption of light and its conversion to heat by the melanin granules in the pigmented epithelium or by photochemical action to the photoreceptor. The focusing effects of the cornea and lens will increase the irradiance on the retina by up to 100,000 times. For visible light 400 to 700 nm, the aversion reflex which takes 0.25 seconds may reduce exposure causing the subject to turn away from a bright light source. However this will not occur if the intensity of the laser is great enough to produce damage in less than 0.25 sec. or when light of 700 - 1400 nm (near infrared) is used as the human eye is insensitive to these wavelengths.[2]

Infrared-B and Infrared-C (1400 to $1.0 \times 10^{+6}$ nm)

Corneal tissue will absorb light with a wavelength longer than 1400 nm. Damage to the cornea results from the absorption of energy by tears and tissue water causing a temperature rise and subsequent denaturation of protein in the corneal surface. Wavelengths from 1400 to 3000 nm penetrate deeper and may lead to the development of cataracts resulting from the heating of proteins in the lens. The critical temperature for damage is not much above normal body temperature.

Laser Radiation Effects on Skin

Skin effects are generally considered of secondary importance except for high power infrared lasers. However with the increased use of lasers emitting in the ultraviolet spectral region, skin effects have assumed greater importance. Erythema (sunburn), skin cancer and accelerated skin aging are produced by emissions in the 200 to 280 nm range. Increased pigmentation results from exposure to light with wavelengths of 280 to 400 nm. Photosensitization has resulted from the skin being exposed to light from 310 to 700 nm. Lasers emitting radiation in the visible and infrared regions produce effects that vary from a mild reddening to blisters and charring. These conditions are usually repairable or reversible however depigmentation, ulceration, and scarring of the skin and damage to underlying organs may occur from extremely high powered lasers.[2]

Summary of Wavelengths of Light and Their Effects on Tissues

Below is a summary of interaction of optical radiation and various tissues. The wavelengths are divided into bands as defied by the International Commission on Illumination (CIE).[2]

CIE band	UV-C	UV-B	UV-A	VISIBLE	IR-A	IR-B	IR-C
	100	280	315	400	700	1400	3000
Adverse effects	Photokeratitis			Retinal Burns		Corneal Burns	
		Cataracts			Cataracts		
	Erythema			Colour Vision Night Vision Degradation			
			Thermal Skin Burns				

Assocaited Hazards
Electrical Hazards

The most lethal hazard associated with lasers is the high voltage electrical systems required to power lasers. Several deaths have occurred when commonly accepted safety practices were not followed by persons working with high voltage sections of laser systems.[2]

Chemical Hazards

Laser Dyes

Most dyes come in a solid powder form, which must be dissolved in solvents prior to use in the laser system. Improper use of dyes or solvents may present a range of hazards for the laser researcher.

Although little is known about them, many organic laser dyes are believed to be toxic and/or mutagenic. Because they are solid powders, they can easily become airborne and be possibly inhaled and/or ingested. When mixed with certain solvents (Dimethylsulphoxide), they can be absorbed through unprotected skin. Direct contact with dyes and with dye/solvent solutions should always be avoided.

A wide variety of solvents are used to dissolve laser dyes. Some of these (alcohols) are highly flammable and must be kept away from ignition sources. Fires and explosions resulting from improper grounding or overheated bearings in dye pumps are not uncommon in laser laboratories. Dye pumps should be inspected, maintained, and tested on a regular basis to avoid these problems. Additionally, dye lasers should never be left running unattended.[2]

Some of the solvents used with laser dyes may also be skin irritants, narcotics, or toxics. One should refer to the Material Safety Data Sheet (MSDS), which is supplied by the solvent manufacturer for additional information on health effects.

Cryogenic Fluids

Cryogenic fluids are used in cooling systems of certain lasers. As these materials evaporate, they replace the oxygen in the air. Adequate ventilation must be ensured. Cryogenic fluids are potentially explosive when ice collects in valves or connectors that are not specifically designed for use with cryogenic fluids. Condensation of oxygen in liquid nitrogen presents a serious explosion hazard if the liquid oxygen comes in contact with any organic material. Although the quantities of liquid nitrogen that are used are small, protective clothing and face shields must be used to prevent freeze burns to the skin and eyes.

Compressed gases used in lasers present serious health and safety hazards. Problems may arise when working with unsecured cylinders, cylinders of hazardous materials not maintained in ventilated enclosures, and gases of different categories (toxins, corrosives, flammable, oxidizers) stored together.[2]

Collateral Radiation

Radiation other than that associated with the primary laser beam is called collateral radiation. Examples are X-rays, UV, plasma, radio frequency emissions.[2]

Ionizing Radiation

X-rays could be produced from two main sources in the laser laboratories. One is high-voltage vacuum tubes of laser power supplies, such as rectifiers, thyratrons and crowbars and the other is electric-discharge lasers. Any power supplies which require more than 15 kilovolts (keV) may produce enough X-rays to cause a health hazard. Interaction between X-rays and human tissue may cause a serious disease such as leukemia or other cancers, or permanent genetic effects which may show up in future generations.[2]

UV and Visible

UV and visible radiation may be generated by laser discharge tubes and pump lamps. The levels produced may exceed the Maximum Permissible Exposure (MPE) and thus cause skin and eye damage.

Plasma Emissions

Interactions between very high power laser beams and target materials may in some instances produce plasmas. The plasma generated may contain hazardous UV emissions.

Radio Frequency (RF)

Q switches (Quality switches) and plasma tubes are RF excited components. Unshielded components may generate radio frequency fields which exceed federal guidelines.[2]

Fire Hazards

Class 4 lasers represent a fire hazard. Depending on construction material beam enclosures, barriers, stops and wiring are all potentially flammable if exposed to high beam irradiance for more than a few seconds.[2]

Explosion Hazards

High pressure arc lamps, filament lamps, and capacitors may explode violently if they fail during operation. These components are to be enclosed in a housing which will withstand the maximum explosive force that may be produced. Laser targets and some optical components also may shatter if heat cannot be dissipated quickly enough. Consequently care must be used to provide adequate mechanical shielding when exposing brittle materials to high intensity lasers.[2]

Laser Accidents

Below is the summary of reported laser accidents in the United States and their causes from 1964 to 1992 (Fig. 16). It indicate that the majority of injuries involve the eye and occur during alignment procedures, or because the protective eyewear was either inappropriate or not used.[2]

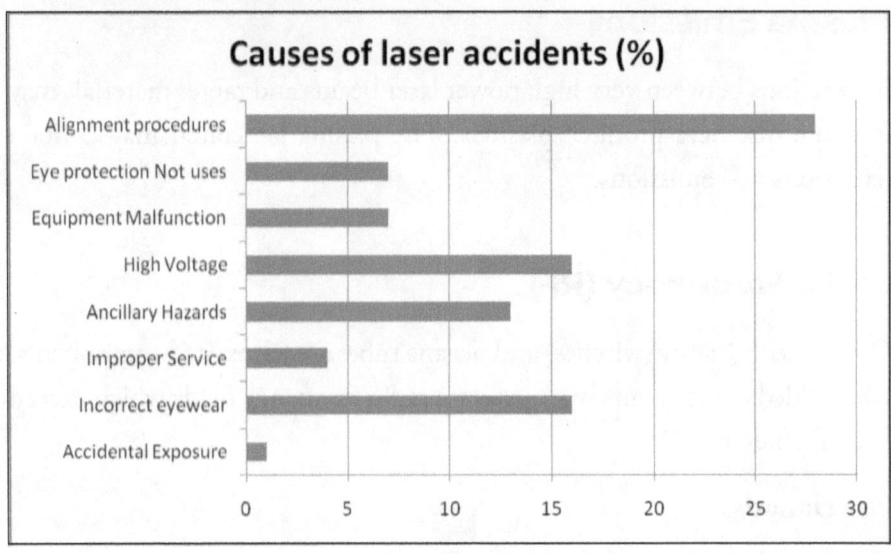

Fig. 16: Causes of laser accidents

LASER SAFETY AND PRECAUTIONS

Patient Safety

The patient is anesthetized or sedated during the surgical procedure. Therefore, the ability of the patient to warn the surgeon of possible injury is impeded or removed. Hence, all efforts for the safety must be directed toward prevention of possible complications. This includes the use of noninflammable materials where possible. Laser resistant shielding materials are available for the surgical field and for protecting the anesthesia equipment. Certain adjustments in the anesthesia technique may also decrease the potential hazards.[6]

Personnel Safety

Personnel working in the laser environment can be at risk for injury. Similar patterns of injury from the laser occur in the workers as in the patients. However, because the operating room personnel are awake, they should be able to be aware of an injury situation that develops. Once aware, they should correct the problem and thereby prevent or minimize the injury.[6]

Absolute rules for the safety of the personnel are as follows:

1. Post signs that lasers are being used. These signs should:
    a. Describe the type of laser.
    b. Indicate the risk class of the laser.
    c. Indicate the required safety equipment for personnel.
    d. State that if unprotected personnel enter the area, the laser is to be turned off.

2. Eye shields must be worn at all times by all personnel.
3. Safety shield must be used.
4. A bucket of sterile water should be immediately available in the operating room.
5. A laser safety officer must be stationed at the laser at all the times.
6. Safety orientation for laser use should be required of all surgeons, anesthesia personnel, and operating room staff.
7. Credentialing of surgeons for use of each type of laser and laser apparatus is needed.

LASER SAFETY CONSIDERATIONS IN DENTISTRY

Properly used by an experienced operator and in a restricted area, the laser is a very safe instrument. The manufacturers have taken great measures to provide a wide margin of safety in the products recommended for dental use, with fail-safe default mechanisms to eliminate accidental exposure (Fig. 17). However, certain safety measures must be strictly adhered to in the dental operatory.[3]

When the laser is in use for any purpose, the access to the operatory should be restricted, a caution sign should be posted and all personnel involved in the treatment, including the patient, must have eye protection (Fig. 18). For the CO_2 laser operation, regular safety glasses with clear lenses are sufficient. The patient should wear safety glasses or have the eyes covered with moist gauze if sedated. The Nd:YAG laser operation requires special dark green lenses for the safety glasses that protect in the blue-green spectrum. Caution should also be taken near reflective surfaces, since the laser beam may be reflected off dental mirrors or instruments and hit other intraoral sites. The innovations in laser equipment laser modified for dental use have significantly reduced the need for a special aiming light with the CO_2 laser, since the flexible wave guide allows a focused beam at 2–4 mm from the target tissue (Luxar Corporation, Bothell, WA). The Nd:YAG laser using the flexible quartz optical fiber in a noncontact mode is also held within a few millimeters of the target tissue. Since the Nd:YAG laser beam is invisible, a coaxial red helium neon laser provides a visible light for the laser (American Dental Laser, Troy, MI). Additional safety standards for fire prevention become necessary when the laser is used in conjunction with general anesthesia and should be reviewed prior to use in the operating room.[3]

Laser vaporous byproducts (laser plume) are generated as smoke once the vaporization of the tissue surface occurs. The plume has been shown to contain particles with mean diameters of 0.1–0.3 pm, and within this plume of carbonized tissue, viable tumor cells and viral particles have been cultured. Animal studies have shown respiratory pathology from laser plume effects to both the CO_2 and Nd:YAG lasers. Baggish et al. have also demonstrated *in vitro* that human immunodeficiency virus (HIV) pro-viral DNA was present in the laser smoke and collected in the evacuation tubing in their laboratory study. Wearing a surgical mask and using high-speed evacuation is essential for infection control, but the standard dental surgical mask does not filter out particles less than 0.5 pm. A new generation of laser surgical masks are now available that will filter to 0.1-pm particles. There are also evacuation systems with filtration for submicron particles that will increase the safety of laser use for biohazardous waste. The Ad Hoc Committee for the American Society for Laser Medicine and Surgery gives the following guidelines concerning hazards of laser plume: 1) all laser personnel should consider the laser plume to be potentially hazardous both in terms of the particulate matter and infectivity, 2) evacuator suction systems with high flow volume and frequent filter changes should be used at all times to collect the plume, the suction tip should be held within 2–5 cm of the laser impact and 3) eye protection, masks, gloves and gowns should be always worn during laser use by all personnel, ensuring that the eyewear protects from splatter, the mask should have good effective filtration and the gloves should preferably be latex.[3]

Laser safety should also include the protection of tooth structure adjacent to the impact site. As mentioned previously in this review, the effects of laser irradiation on enamel or root surfaces can be detrimental when the focused mode is used for soft tissue ablation. Placing a periodontal retractor between the tooth and gingiva while attempting to hit the surface at a 90° angle will afford the best protection during soft tissue removal.[3]

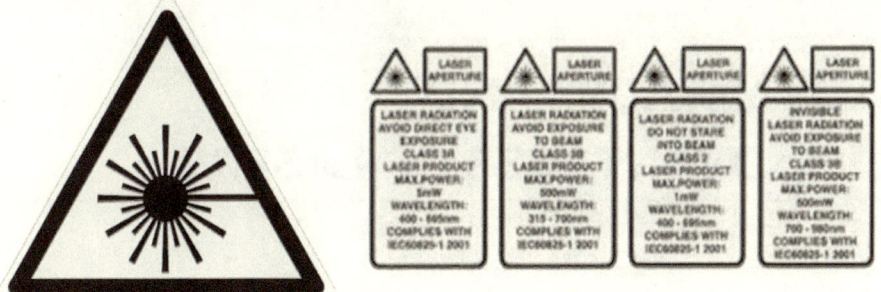

Fig. 17: Types of laser safety signs and labels

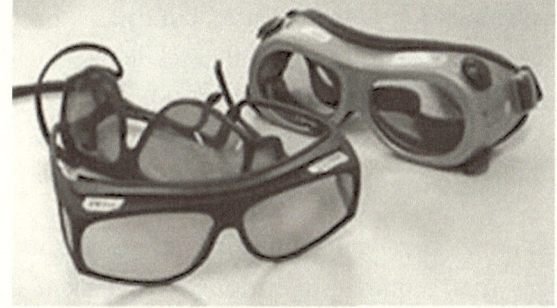

Fig 18: Protective eyeglasses used for different lasers depending on the wavelength of the laser beam

ADVANTAGES AND DISADVANTAGES OF LASERS

Advantages of laser treatment in periodontics are effective and efficient soft and hard tissue ablation with a greater hemostasis, bactericidal effect, minimal wound contraction, minimal collateral damages with reduced use of local analgesia. In addition, the small popping sound of the lasers in action with Er:YAG seems to produce less stress to patients than the high pitch vibration sound of most of the ultrasonic devices.[92]

Despite numerous advantages of using lasers, the use of laser also has disadvantages that require precautions to be taken during clinical application. Laser irradiation can interact with tissues even in the non-contact mode, which means that laser beams may reach the patient's eye and other tissues surrounding the target in the oral cavity. Clinicians should be careful to prevent inadvertent irradiation to these tissues, especially to the eyes. Protective eyewear specific for the wavelength of the laser in use must be worn by patient, operator, and assistant.[92]

It is recommended that dental laser users to attend certification courses provided by some dental laser organizations and follow laser safety guidelines such as the Laser Code of Practice from the Hong Kong Surgical Laser Association. A good understanding in laser wavelength characteristics, tissue interaction and laser device specification provide a platform for achieving the best results.[92]

Finally, the cost and size of laser device still constitute an obstacle for clinical application of the lasers. Laser device like Er:YAG and Er,Cr:YSGG are usually cumbersome and rather difficult to set up in small dental surgeries in several countries.

SUMMARY AND CONCLUSION

Lasers have been suggested as an adjunctive or alternative to conventional techniques for various dental procedures and considered superior in respect to easy ablation, decontamination, and hemostasis along with less operative and post-operative pain. Introduction of lasers in implant therapy and newer laser technical modalities has revolutionised the periodontal treatment outcome with patient acceptance. Laser Assisted Periodontal Therapy is non-invasive. With diode laser there is a reduced need for systemic or locally applied antimicrobials. This leads to fewer allergic reactions and antibiotic resistance.

Given the incredible ease of use and its versatility in treating soft tissue, the diode laser becomes the "soft tissue handpiece" in the dentist's armamentarium. The dentists can use the laser handpiece to remove, refine and adjust soft tissues in the same way that the traditional dental handpiece is used on enamel and dentin. This extends the scope of practice of the general dentist to include many soft tissue procedures. The patient's gingival health is improved in a minimally invasive, gentler manner.

On the other side, cost, safety issues, technical complexities, and lack of evidence-based studies about therapeutic effects and efficiencies are drawbacks of laser treatment. The erbium group lasers appear to be the choice laser in periodontics.

We have to take into account that laser treatments are in continuous evolution; possibly in the upcoming years our scope will be to have equipments combining different photonic properties allowing us to choose the most adequate system for each necessity. Although there has been a great progress in the past few years, most of the studies are difficult to be evaluated clinically, due to their short duration (2 to 3 months). More long term systematic studies are necessary to evaluate the clinical and biological effects of each type of laser, the time and application mode, unique/multiple doses and application frequency. It will also be essential to know the appropriate energies of each kind of laser. Application comfort, the silence, anesthesia reduction and other such advantages make lasers attractive for society and professionals.

REFERENCES

1. **Vivek K Bains, Sanjay Gupta and Rhythm Bains.** *Lasers in Periodontics: An Overview.* 2010, Journal of Oral Health Community Dentistry, Vol. 4 (spl).
2. Lasers. *Wikipedia.* [Online] en.wikipedia.org/wiki/Laser.
3. **Jeffrey A. Rossmann and Charles M. Cobb.** *Lasers in periodontal therapy.* 1995, Periodontology 2000, Vol. 9, pp. 150–164. 0906–6713.
4. **Babu Mathew and Prasanth S.** *LASERS IN DENTISTRY.* 2, Jul-Dec -2011, Oral & Maxillofacial Pathology Journal, Vol. 2. 0976–1225.
5. **Csele, Mark.** *Fundamentals of Light Sources and Lasers.* s.l. : Wiley Interscience, 2004.
6. **Guy A. Catone and Charles C. Alling.** *Laser Applications in Oral and Maxillofacial Surgery.* s.l. : W.B. Saunders, 1997.
7. **AKIRA AOKI, et al.** *Lasers in nonsurgical periodontal therapy.* 2004, Periodontology 2000, Vol. 36, pp. 59–97.
8. **Neetha, et al.** *Dental Lasers.* 2, 2010, Journal of Dental Science, Vol. 1.
9. **Hennig T, Rechmann P and Spengler B.** *Selective ablation of subgingival calculus.* Singapore : s.n., 1994, 4th International Congress on Lasers in Dentistry, p. 11.
10. **RL, Finkbeiner.** *The results of 1328 periodontal pockets treated with the argon laser: Selective pocket thermolysis.* 1995, J Clin Laser Med Surg, Vol. 13, pp. 273–281.

11. **Israel M and Rossman JA.** *An epithelian exclusion technique using the CO_2 laser for the treatment of periodontal defects.* 1998, Compendium, Vol. 19, pp. 86, 88, 90, 92–95.
12. **K, Ishikawa.** *Effects of Nd: YAG laser irradiation in the periodontal pockets on bacterial adhesion and change of temperature on root surfaces and clinical symptoms.* 1996, Aichi-Gakuin J Dent Sci, Vol. 34, pp. 465–480.
13. **M, Luomanen.** *Oral focal epithelian hyperplasia removed with CO_2 laser.* 1990, Int J Oral Maxillofac Surg, Vol. 19, pp. 205–207.
14. **M, Luomanen.** *The use of CO_2 laser surgery for removal of multiple oral epithelian hyperplasias.* 1989, Proc Finn Dent Soc, Vol. 85, pp. 41–46.
15. **JW, Frame.** *Carbon dioxide laser surgery for benign oral lesions.* 1985, Br Dent J, Vol. 158, pp. 125–128.
16. **Hattler AB, Kirschner RA and Susanin PB.** *Laser surgery for immunosuppressive gingival hyperplasia.* 1992, Periodont Clin Invest, Vol. 14, pp. 18–20.
17. **Convissar RA, Diamond LB and Fazekas CDL.** *Laser treatment of orthodontically induced gingival hyperplasia.* 1996, Gen Dent, Vol. 44, pp. 47–51.
18. **SR, Epstein.** *The frenectomy: A comparison of classic versus laser technique.* 1991, Pract Periodont Aesthet Dent, Vol. 3, pp. 27–31.
19. **Gelskey SC, White JM and Pruthi VK.** *The effectiveness of the Nd: YAG laser in the treatment of dental hypersensitivity.* 1993, J Can Dent Assoc, Vol. 59, pp. 377–378, 383–386.
20. **Gerschman JA, Ruben J and Gebart-Eaglemont J.** *Low level laser therapy for dentinal tooth hypersensitivity.* 1994, Aust Dent J, Vol. 39, pp. 353–357, .
21. **Gutknecht N, Moritz A and Dercks HW.** *Treatment of hypersensitive teeth using neodymium:yttrium-aluminum-garnet lasers: A comparison of the use of various settings in an in vivo study.* 1997, J Clin Laser Med Surg, Vol. 15, pp. 171–174.

22. **Bass LS and Treat MR.** *Laser tissue welding: A comprehensive review of current and future clinical applications.* 1995, Lasers Surg Med, Vol. 17, pp. 315–349.
23. **Pecaro B and Garehime W.** *The CO_2 laser in oral maxillofacial surgery.* 1983, J Oral Maxillofac Surg, Vol. 41, pp. 725–728.
24. **JH, Rice.** *Laser-assisted second stage recovery of implants.* 1996, Wavelengths, Vol. 4, pp. 6–7.
25. **Centty I G, Blank L W and Levy B A.** *Carbon dioxide laser for de-epithelialization of periodontal flaps.* 1997, J Periodontol, Vol. 68, pp. 763–769.
26. **Olivi G, Crippa R, Iaria G, Kaitsas V, DiVito E, Stefano B.** Laser in endodontics. Endodontic International 2011; 7(1): 1-7.
27. http://www.dentaltribune.com/articles/specialities/endodontics/5491_laser_in_endodontic s_part_i.html. Accessed on 10.02.2015.
28. **Sathe S, Hegde V, Jain PA, Ghunawat D.** Effectiveness of Er: YAG (PIPS) and Nd: YAG activation on final irrigants for smear layer removal - SEM observation. Journal of Dental Lasers 2014; 8(1): 8-13.
29. **OliviG, DiVitoE.** Photoacoustic Endodontics using PIPS™: experimental background and clinical protocol. Journal of the Laser and Health Academy 2012; 1: 22-5.
30. **Mohammed SA, Enrico D, Christopher VH, Dan N, George TH.** Photomedicine and Laser Surgery 2014; 32(5): 260-6.
31. **Coluzzi DJ.** Fundamentals of lasers in dentistry basic science tissue interaction and instrumentation. J laser Dent 2008;16:4-10.
32. **Schoop U, Kluger W, Moritz A Nedjelik N, Georgopoulos A, Sperr W.** Bactericidal effect of different laser systems in the deep layers of dentin. Lasers in Surgery and Medicine 2004; 35(2): 111-16.
33. Proceedings of the 1st International Workshop of Evidence Based Dentistry on Lasers in Dentistry, Quintessence Publishing, 2007, ISBN 978-1-85097-167-2.

34. **Gutknecht N, Franzen R, Lampert F.** Finite Element Study on Thermal Effects in Root Canals During Laser Treatment with a Surface-absorbed Laser. Lasers Med Sci 2002; 17: 137-44.
35. **Blöschl G, Kirnbauer R, Gutknecht D.** Distributed snowmelt simulations in an Alpine catchment. 1. Model evaluation on the basis of snow cover patterns. Water Resources Research 1991; 27(12): 3171-9.
36. **Gutknecht N, Moritz A, Conrads G, Sievert T, Lampert F.** Bactericidal effect of the Nd: YAG laser in in vitro root canals. J Clin Laser Med Surg 1996; 14: 77-80.
37. **Rooney J, Midda M, Leeming J.** A laboratory investigation of the bactericidal effect of a Nd:YAG laser. Br Dent Journal 1994; 22: 61-4.
38. **Hardie EM, Stone EA, Spaulding KA, Cullen JM.** Subtotal canine prostatectomy with the neodymium: yttrium-aluminium-garnet laser. Vet Surg 1990; 19(5): 348-55.
39. **Klinke T, Klimm W, Gutknecht N.** Antibacterial effects of the Nd:YAG laser irradiation within root canal dentin. J Clin Med Surg 1997; 15: 29-31.
40. **Orstavik D, Haapasalo M.** Disinfection by endodontic irrigants and dressings of experimentally infected dentinal tubules. Endodontics and Dental Traumatology 1990; 6: 142-9.
41. **Gutknecht N.** Lasers in Endodontics. Journal of the Laser and Health Academy 2008; 4: 1-8.
42. **Mathew S, Thangaraj DN.** Lasers In Endodontics. JIADS 2010; 1(1): 31-7.
43. **Gorkhay K.** Effects of oral soft tissue produced by a diode laser in vitro. Lasers in Surgery and Medicine.1999; 25: 401-6.
44. **Lee BS.** Ultra structural changes of human dentin after irradiation by Nd:YAG laser. Lasers Surg Med 2002: 30(3): 246-52.
45. **Pozza DH, Fregapani PW, Xavier CB, Weber JB, Oliviera MG.** CO_2, Er:YAG and ND:YAG lasers in endodontic surgery. J appl Oral Sci 2009; 17(6): 596-9.

46. **Neville BW, Damm DD, Allen CM, et al.** Oral and maxillofacial pathology: 3rd ed. St. Louis: Saunders Elsevier; 2008.
47. **Catone GA, Alling CC.** Laser applications in oral and maxillo facial surgery 1st ed. Philadelphia: WB Saunders; 1997.
48. **Ossoff RH, Coleman JA, Courey MS, et al.** Clinical application of laser in otolaryngology—head and neck surgery. Lasers Surg Med 1994; 15(3): 217-248.
49. **Siegel MA.** Diagnosis and management of recurrent herpes simplex infections. J Am Dental Assoc 2002; 133(9): 1245-1249.
50. **De Souza To, Martins MA, Bussadori SK, et al.** Clinical evaluation of low-level laser treatment for recurring aphthous stomatitis. Phtomed Laser Surg 2010 Oct; 282(2): 85-88.
51. **Walsh LJ.** The current status of low level laser therapy in dentistry. Part 1 Soft tissue applications. Australian Dent J 1997; 42(4): 247-254.
52. **Walsh LJ.** The current status of low level laser therapy in dentistry. Part 2 Hard tissue applications. Australian Dent J 1997; 42(5): 302-306.
53. **Bayer DB, Stenger TG.** 'Trigeminal neuralgia: an overview'. Oral Surg Oral Med Oral Pathol 1979; 48(5): 393-399.
54. Headache Classification Committee of the International Headache Society. The international classification of head ache disorders. Cephalalgia 2004; 24(1): 1-160.
55. **Eckerdal A, Bastin L.** Can low reactive-level laser therapy be used in treatment of neurogenic facial pain? A double blind placebo controlled investigation of patients with trigeminal neuralgia. Laser Ther 1996; 8: 247-252.
56. **Eckerdal A, Bastin L.** A double blind placebo controlled investigation of patients with trigeminal neuralgia. Laser Ther 2003; 12: 112-120.
57. **Dundar U, Ericke D, Samli F, et al.** The effect of Gallium laser therapy in the management of myofacial pain syndrome. Clin Rheumathol 2007; 26(6): 930-934.

58. **Bradly P, Heller G.** The effect of 830 nm laser on chronic myofacial pain. Pain 2006; 124(1-2): 201-210.
59. **Shirani AM, Gutknecht N, Taghizadeh M, Mir M.** Low level laser therapy and myofacial pain dysfunction syndrome: a randomized controlled clinical trial. Lasers Med Sci 2009; 24(5): 715-720.
60. **Dworkin SF, LeResche L.** Research diagnostic criteria for temporomandibular disorders: review, criteria, examinations and specifications, critique. J Craniomandib Disord 1992; 6(4): 301-355.
61. **Rollmann GB, Gillespie JM.** The role of psychosocial factors in temporomandibular disorders. Curr Rev Pain 2000; 4(1): 71-81.
62. **Bertolucci LE, Grey T.** Clinical analysis of mid-laser versus placebo treatment of arthralgic TMJ degenerative joints. J Craniomand Prac 1995; 13(1): 26-29.
63. **De Abreu Venancio R, Camparis CM, De Fátima Zantirato, et al.** Low intensity laser therapy in the treatment of temporo mandibular disorders: a double-blind study. J Oral Rehabil 2005; 32(11): 800-807.
64. **Huang TC, Dalton JB, Monsour FN, Savage NW.** Multiple, large sialoliths of the submandibular gland duct: a case report. Aust Dent J 2009; 54(1): 61-65.
65. **Ergun S, Mete O, Yeşil S, Tanyeri H.** Solitary angiokeratoma of the tongue treated with Diode Laser. Lasers Med Sci 2009; 24(4): 123-125.
66. **Pick RM, Colvard MD.** Current status of lasers in soft tissue dental surgery. J Periodontol 1993;64(7):589-602.
67. **Kopp WK, St-Hilaire H.** Mucosal preservation in the treatment of mucocele with CO_2 laser. J Oral Maxillofac Surg 2004; 62(12): 1559-1561.
68. **Mota-Ramírez A, Javier Silvestre F, Simó JM.** Oral biopsy in dental practice. Med Oral Patol Oral Cir Bucal 2007; 2(7): E504-510.
69. **Bornstein MM, Winzap-Kälin C, Cochran DL, Buser D.** The CO_2 laser for excisional biopsies of oral lesions: a case

series study. Int J Periodontics Restorative Dent 2005; 5(3): 221-229.
70. **Brantley WA, Eliades T.** Orthodontic Materials. Stuttgart: Thieme; 2001.
71. **Von Fraunhofer JA, Allen DJ, Orbell GM.** Laser etching of enamel for direct bonding. Angle Orthod 1993; 63: 73-6.
72. **Strobl K, Bahns TL, Willham L, Bishara SE, Stwalley WC.** Laser-aided debonding of orthodontic ceramic brackets. Am J Orthod Dentofacial Orthop 1992; 101: 152-8.
73. **Talbot TQ, Blankenau RJ, Zobitz ME, Weaver AL, Lohse CM, Rebellato J.** Effect of argon laser irradiation on shear bond strength of orthodontic brackets: An in vitro study. Am J Orthod Dentofacial Orthop 2000; 118: 274-9.
74. **Graber TM, Vanarsdall RL.** Current Principles and Techniques in Orthodontics. St. Louis: Mosby-Year Book; 1994.
75. **Smith TA, Thompson JA, Lee WE.** Assessing patient pain during dental laser treatment. J Am Dent Assoc 1993; 124: 90-5.
76. **Lim HM, Lew KK, Tay DK.** A clinical investigation of the efficacy of low level laser therapy in reducing orthodontic postadjustment pain. Am J Orthod Dentofacial Orthop 1995; 108: 614-22.
77. **Corpas-Pastor L, Villalba Moreno J, de Dios Lopez-Gonzalez Garrido J, Pedraza Muriel V, Moore K, Elias A.** Comparing the tensile strength of brackets adhered to laser-etched enamel vs. acid-etched enamel. J Am Dent Assoc 1997; 128: 732-7.
78. **Rickabaugh JL, Marangoni RD, McCaffrey KK.** Ceramic bracket debonding with the carbon dioxide laser. Am J Orthod Dentofacial Orthop 1996; 110: 388-93.
79. **Kurchak M, DeSantos B, Powers J, Turner D.** Argon laser for light-curing adhesives. J Clin Orthod 1997; 31: 371-4.
80. **Lee BS, Hsieh TT, Lee YL, Lan WH, Hsu YJ, Wen PH, et al.** Bond strengths of orthodontic bracket after acid-etched, Er: YAG laser-irradiated and combined treatment on enamel surface. Angle Orthod 2003; 73: 565-70.

81. **Weinberger SJ, Foley TF, McConnell RJ, Wright GZ.** Bond strengths of two ceramic brackets using argon laser, light, and chemically cured resin systems. Angle Orthod 1997; 67: 173-8.
82. **Tocchio RM, Williams PT, Mayer FJ, Standing KG.** Laser debonding of ceramic orthodontic brackets. Am J Orthod Dentofacial Orthop 1993; 103: 155-62.
83. **Miserendino L.J. Pick R.M.,** Lasers in dentistry. Chicago. Quintessence Publishing. 1995; 133-68.
84. **Eduardo CP.,** the state of the Art of lasers in esthetic and Prosthodontics. J Oral Laser Applications 2005; 5: 135-143.
85. **Parker S.,** Lasers and soft tissues: – fixed' soft tissue surgery. Br Dent J. 2007; 202: 247-53.
86. **Manni J.G.,** Dental applications of advanced lasers, Barlington(VT). JGM associates. 1996.
87. **Strauss R.,** Lasers in oral and maxillofacial surgery. Dent Clin N Am. 2000; 44(4): 861-88.
88. **Kato T., Kusakari H., Hoshino E.,** Bactericidal efficacy of carbon dioxide laser against bacteria-contaminated titanium implant and subsequent cellular adhesion to irradiated area. Lasers Surg Med. 1998; 23(5): 299–309.
89. **Jeusette M.** The floating ridge the thickened arch: a necessary evil? Rev Belge Med Dent. 1999; 54: 61-9.
90. **Kimura Y, Yu DG, Fujita A, Yamashita A, Murakami Y, Matsumoto K.,** Effects of erbium, chromium:YSGG laser irradiation on canine mandibular bone. J Periodonto. 2001; 72: 1178–82.
91. **Ramya J.** et al., Lasers in Prosthetic dentistry. Indian Journal of applied Research 2013; 3(4): 369-370.
92. **Lee, Dae-hyun.** *Application of Laser in Periodontics: A New Approach in Periodontal Treatment.* 10, s.l. : Dental Bulletin, 2007, Vol. 12.

www.ingramcontent.com/pod-product-compliance
Lightning Source LLC
Chambersburg PA
CBHW020921180526
45163CB00007B/2829